Vital Nutrition

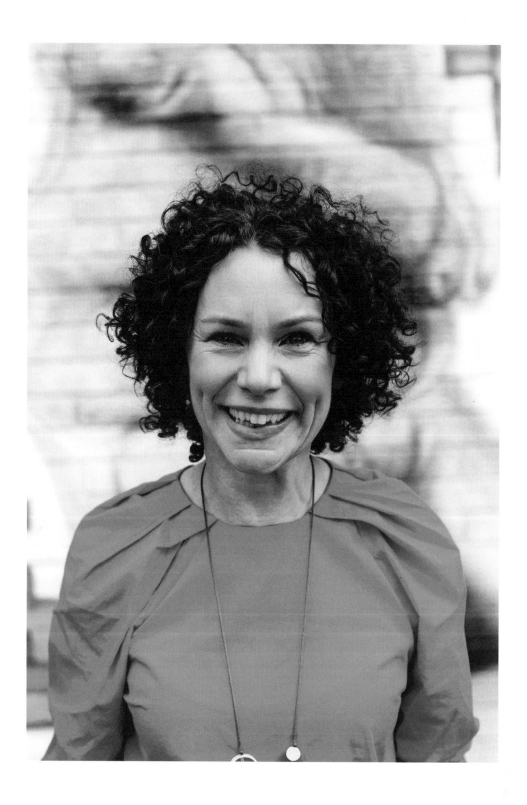

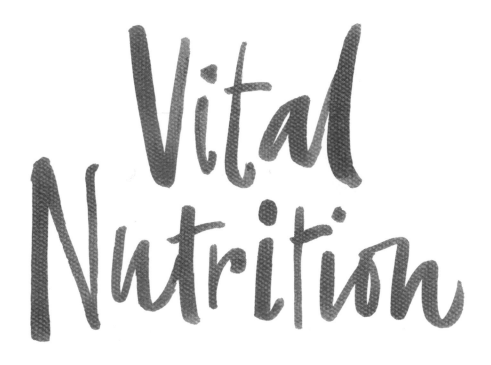

Vital Nutrition

How to eat for optimum health, happiness and energy

JANE McCLENAGHAN

·THE·
BLACK
·STAFF·
PRESS

To all the people I have been fortunate enough to work with over the years,
who show me the power of nutrition in real life every day.

First published in 2017 by Blackstaff Press, part of Colourpoint Creative
Colourpoint House
Jubilee Business Park
21 Jubilee Road
Newtownards BT23 4YH

Designed by seagulls.net
Printed in Antrim by W. & G. Baird

ISBN 978 0 85640 991 2

www.blackstaffpress.com
www.vital-nutrition.co.uk
www.martina-scott.com

Follow Jane on Twitter @vitalnutrition

Some names and identifying details have been changed
to protect the privacy of individuals.

Although every effort has been made to ensure that the contents of this
book are accurate, it must not be treated as a substitute for qualified
medical advice. Always consult a qualified medical practitioner.
Neither the author nor the publisher can be held responsible
for any loss or claim arising out of the use or misuse of the
suggestions made or the failure to take medical advice.

Contents

Acknowledgements

A great big thank you to Helen Wright and Patsy Horton at Blackstaff Press for their hard work, enthusiasm and encouragement. Thanks to Martina Scott for the beautiful images she has created to help bring the book to life and to Jess Lowe for her quirky photographic skills. To Susie Perry for her keen eye and nutritional knowledge.

Thank you to everyone in the Vital Nutrition Book Club for their contributions to the book. I loved your input and inspirational ideas.

Finally, thank you to the very important people in my life – Nev, my Mum & Dad, Aaron, Vickie, Bethan, Owen and Sam. You rock!

Introduction

As a nutritional therapist, I am passionate about the amazing effects that good food has on our health and wellbeing. Over the years I have seen hundreds of people turn their health around, thanks to the power of food.

We do not have to go to extremes to benefit from good nutrition. A few simple changes that you can stick with long term are much more beneficial to your health than any crazy diet. I think most of us do our best to eat as well as we can, but sometimes we need a little encouragement or some new ideas to enthuse us about healthy eating again.

Rather than clearing out our cupboards to make way for weird and wonderful foods, we can all make some simple changes to what we put in our shopping baskets to improve our diet and health. Wellness starts with the food we have in our larders and fridges, as that is what ends up on our plates. We can literally eat our way to better health, improved vitality and a feeling of wellness.

In this book I have brought together the key ideas and principles of nutrition, based on the latest research, to inspire you to connect to the food on your plate and use it as your daily wellbeing tonic. Although there is no such thing as a 'one-size-fits-all' approach to nutrition, there are a few principles from which all of us can benefit.

In my clinic and workshops I work with people who are seeking an effective way of taking responsibility for their health and wellbeing. When I was writing this book, some of these clients came together to form the Vital Nutrition Book Club, to share ideas of what works for them. Between us, we came up with a list of the most common questions and queries people have about diet and nutrition to make the advice given in this book as useful and practical as possible. You will find stories and comments from the Book Club members throughout this book.

When writing this book I wanted to gather together all the most useful and important information and tips I have learned over the years to set out a way of eating that will bring you optimum health, happiness and energy. So whether you have a burning interest in all things healthy, or are just dipping your toe in the field of nutrition, I hope that you will find ideas to inspire you to make positive, nutritious changes for the good of your health. This is real-life nutrition. Remember, it's the simple things that make the difference.

Chapter One
How Healthy Are You?

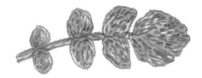

What we eat

No matter what your age or stage of life, it is never too late to start making changes to what you buy, cook and eat with a view to maximising your potential to feel and look your very best.

Study after study tells us that we can eat our way to better health, showing that we can reduce our risk of developing conditions like cardiovascular disease, type 2 diabetes and cancer. So if we know all this, then why is it so damn hard to eat a healthy diet?

Put simply, the answer is that we are human! We are creatures of habit, we eat in reaction to our emotions, and we have funny food aversions and associations. If all it took was understanding the basics of nutrition, then we would all be eating nourishing, healthy food and never crave chocolate, yearn for fast-food takeaways or need a second helping of dessert.

Of course food is much more than just the sum of its nutrients. We eat to socialise, we comfort eat, we binge eat, we eat because there is something tasty in the fridge, we eat with friends … Food is a beautiful way of bringing people together. Most of us connect with family and friends over food, whether it's Sunday dinner, a Friday night out with mates or lunchtime meet-ups. Food is social, food is comforting, food

1

is fuel; food can be your friend or food can be your foe. Do you relish every morsel and see food as a celebration of life, or do you feel fear and guilt with every bite you take? Most of us have a love–hate relationship with food. We have become so far removed from the process of growing, cooking and eating food that we dash into the supermarket, buy convenience food that promises to save us time and effort, and then wolf it down without much thought as to the effects it has on our health.

If you would like to make some positive changes to your diet and health, then a great starting point is to think about your relationship with food. What does food mean to you? Once we can build a more positive relationship with the food on our plate, our health is almost certain to benefit.

Here are some ideas from my family, friends and clients to get you thinking.

Food is ...

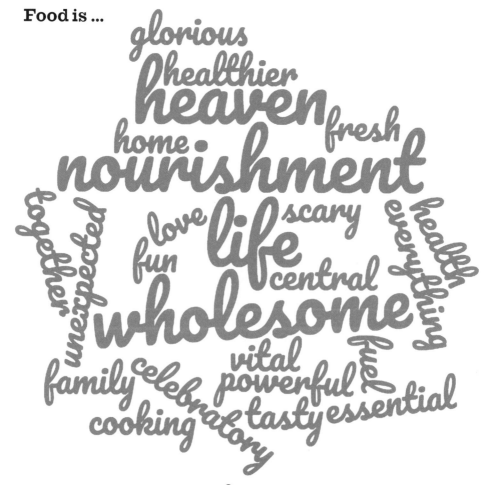

Over 2,500 years ago, Hippocrates – the father of modern medicine – said, 'Let food be thy medicine and medicine be thy food.' His statement holds true today. With the NHS in crisis, obesity, heart disease and cancer on the increase and risk of type 2 diabetes at record levels, we need to take responsibility for our health. Let food be your medicine and give yourself the best possible chance of a good-health day every day!

The truth behind the headlines

Thanks to social media, advertising, newspapers and magazines, we are surrounded by images of food. We are constantly being offered advice about what, when and how to eat by Instagrammers, TV chefs and news headlines. How do we sort the truth from the nonsense and find out what a healthy diet really looks (and tastes) like?

My years of working as a nutritional therapist have confirmed my belief that we need to get back to basics and reconnect with the effects the food on our plate has on our health.

I come from a family that has farmed for at least the last five generations – my uncle and cousins are still farming – whose livelihood was intertwined with the seasons, who knew the impact of good food, and who had a belief in the healing properties of plants and nature. I am sure that my farming background sparked my interest in food – it certainly gave me the belief that if we are in tune with how food makes us feel and notice the changes that good nutrition makes to our health and wellbeing, then eating well is not a struggle or chore but instead a way of connecting with our bodies, nourishing our minds and managing our health.

What is a healthy diet?

Eat a low-fat diet. Eat more protein. Go Paleo. Cut out sugar. Count calories. Fast twice a week. There is a maze of nutritional advice out there. Finding our way through it is tricky and can leave us feeling confused, guilty and stressed. There is so much conflicting advice around that it's really hard to understand the best way to eat. So how do you know what is right for your body and what a healthy, balanced diet really looks like?

If you've tried every new eating plan, spent your adult life yo-yo dieting and are still on a rollercoaster, feeling scared by food and its effects on your body, then this book can help to show you a better way of eating that is nourishing, healthful and positive.

One size does not fit all, which is why a diet that works for your friends can make you feel ravenous, exhausted or miserable. We are all different, with different genetic make-ups, different lifestyles, different tastes, different likes and different dislikes. Foods that are good for your health may not suit me – the idea that there is one diet out there that will suit all of us is a myth.

Once we really connect with how our body uses the food we eat and the impact that food has on how we think and feel, the need to be controlling about food starts to vanish. I want to share some insider knowledge so that you have a real understanding of the powerful effects that food has on your wellbeing – that it is much more than just calories, and instead is a source of energy and vitality in the form of textures, flavours and colours, providing us with vitamins, minerals, phytonutrients, amino acids, energy, fats and fibre to nourish our body from the inside out.

You are one of a kind!

As humans we have complex nutritional needs which change depending on our age and stage of life, our genetics and family history, and our level of activity and exercise. All humans have the same basic need for good, balanced nutrition. If we can get the foundations right, then we can start to change and adapt the building blocks that go on top according to our own individual needs. This enables us to create a bespoke diet.

We are living in an exciting time in which individualised nutrition is possible thanks to advances in genetics and nutritional science. A new and emerging area of scientific research called epigenetics could change the way we look at diet, nutrition and lifestyle in the future. In the next decade there promises to be a food revolution like never before as the study of the human genome and the impact that our diet and lifestyle has on our own very individual biochemistry is revealed.

What do you eat?

Is your plate well balanced and packed full of goodness, or is something missing? Our bodies need a complete balance of nutrition to function at their very best. If we neglect any of the nutrient groups for a few days we should continue to function fine – the body can adjust and reset the balance – but if this goes on for weeks, months, or years, then our bodies will start to send out a cry for help.

Cravings, skin eruptions, IBS, bad breath, mood swings, white spots on fingernails – these are all possible signs that your body is missing nutrients. Every cell in our bodies needs good nutrition. We are made of the nutrients in the food we eat. Wow! That is mind-blowing, isn't it? The microscopic cells that make up our hair, immune system, gut lining, brain cells and all the other cells are made using the food we eat. If we leave out any food group or eat too much of another, we throw our delicate nutritional balance out of sync. For optimal health and wellbeing we need to nourish our body from the inside out.

What we need to eat

Here are the key nutrients your body needs not just to survive, but also to thrive.

Protein

Found in eggs, meat, fish, chicken, nuts, seeds, pulses, dairy foods, protein is constructed from little building blocks called amino acids. These amino acids in turn become the building blocks for proteins in your body that provide structure, communication and sparks to ignite and regulate functions of the body, for example, collagen to keep your skin supple, insulin for blood sugar balance, haemoglobin to transport iron, amylase to break down carbohydrates. All of these substances and substrates are built using amino acids that originate from the protein on our plate.

Garlic

Superfoods

Garlic has been heralded as a superfood since medieval times. Renowned for its benefits for heart health, liver support, antimicrobial effects and cancer prevention, this common ingredient is a key food for health.

To make the most of your garlic, crush or chop it to stimulate the conversion of alliin into the beneficial allicin. Once crushed or chopped, leave it for a couple of minutes to let the conversion happen and then eat – once the garlic is cut, it loses its potency very quickly and most of the allicin will disappear within about an hour. If you cook with garlic, add it towards the end of cooking to maximise the benefits.

Garlic that comes ready chopped, dried or powdered does not have the same benefits.

Fat

Thanks to crazy low-fat diets, calorie counting and diet restriction, fat has been the neglected macronutrient in our diets since the 1970s. It had a reputation as being high calorie, making us fat, increasing cholesterol and generally being the bad guy of nutrition, but fat is making a comeback. We now know how important omega-3 and -6 fats, monounsaturated fats and even some saturated fats are for our health. Without fat in our diet it would be virtually impossible to absorb vitamins A, D, E and K, not to mention the masses of fat-soluble antioxidants like carotenoids and CoQ10. Eaten in moderation, fat does not make us fat, and neither does it increase cholesterol. It is an extremely valuable nugget of nutrition for your body and is used to:

- help regulate inflammation
- support healthy metabolism
- contribute to normal skin hydration
- protect your cells
- carry fat-soluble vitamins
- contribute to the regulation of hormone balance
- support healthy neurotransmitter balance
- help regulate appetite

What's not to love? Get more good fat into your diet by eating more of these foods:

- oily fish (sardines, mackerel, herring, trout, salmon)
- nuts (walnuts, almonds, macadamia nuts, Brazil nuts)
- seeds (sunflower, pumpkin, sesame, flax, chia)
- olive oil (for dressings, drizzles and cooking at lower temperatures)
- coconut oil (for cooking at higher temperatures)
- avocado
- tahini

Carbohydrate

Carbohydrate is used for energy. Full stop. That's it. Nothing else. Like every other nutrient, carbohydrate is essential, it's just a case of finding a healthy balance. Choosing complex carbohydrates – like wholegrain cereals, legumes and root vegetables – provides us with a slow, sustained energy source packed with additional vitamins and minerals that are essential to our health, while the refined and processed simple carbohydrates and sugary foods are devoid of much nutritional value.

Vitamins and minerals

The A to Z of essential vitamins and minerals have a huge range of jobs to do in your body, and although available as nutritional supplements, the best place to start is a balanced, varied diet.

Apples

An apple a day could help with weight loss, reduce risk of type 2 diabetes, balance cholesterol and improve our brain health. Packed with antioxidant bioflavonoids and fibre, apples also appear to have prebiotic effects thanks to their high pectin content.

Superfoods

Fibre

Fibre keeps your digestion in good nick and bowel movements regular. Sources of fibre, like wholegrain cereals, nuts, seeds, fruit and vegetables, also help to slow the release of sugar (or energy) from food, so we get a steady, sustained release rather than a quick surge. Fibre also plays a role in balancing the good gut bacteria of our microbiome and keeping those little gut bugs happy, balanced and healthy.

Water

Water hydrates cells, regulates digestion and helps keep your skin clear. Most advice states that we should have 1.5 to 2 litres of water every day and this can include herbal teas, but not regular tea, coffee, juice or fizzy drinks.

So what should be on our plates?

So if these are the key nutrients we need, let's take a look at how we fit them together to make a healthy, balanced diet.

In 2015 BANT (The British Association for Applied Nutrition and Nutritional Therapy) launched its Wellness Solution Plate based on up-to-date research – providing easy to understand, meaningful information to help us strike a healthy balance on our plates.

One of the first things you will notice about the Wellness Solution Plate is that vegetables make up the main proportion of the food we should be eating – leafy greens, root veg and other veg. When it comes to our vegetable choices, not all

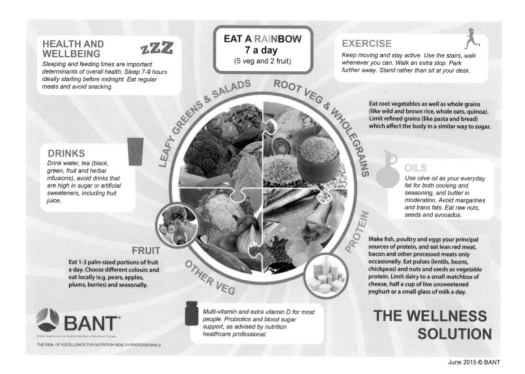

June 2015 © BANT

vegetables are created equal. Notice that a quarter of the plate consists of leafy greens and salad. These nutritional powerhouses are packed with essential nutrients including magnesium, folic acid and iron. Other vegetables like onions, peppers, cauliflower and peas add variety on the next quarter of your plate, and root vegetables are included in the carbohydrate choices alongside wholegrains like brown rice, oats and quinoa. For years government advice stated that we should eat 'plenty of bread, rice, potatoes and pasta'. The Wellness Solution Plate highlights the fact that refined grains affect our bodies in a similar way to sugar and should be limited.

You may be surprised to see that these new recommendations suggest we should be eating no more than two portions of fruit a day – this is to limit our sugar intake. Choosing fruit that grows locally is not only better for our environment, thanks to reduced food miles, but is better for us too. Tropical fruit – like pineapples, mangos and bananas – tends to be higher in natural sugars than the fruit that grows in our climate – apples, pears, plums, berries and cherries. On that note, eat your fruit, don't drink it. Every glass of juice you drink contains as much sugar as a glass of fizzy pop. When we eat the whole fruit rather than drink its juice, we have the benefit of fibre to slow down the sugar release. One glass of juice can contain two to four portions

Your Daily Wellness Plate

Your breakfast plate

2 scrambled eggs (protein) with spinach (leafy greens), tomato (other veg) and toasted rye bread (wholegrains).

OR

Jumbo porridge oats (wholegrains) with berries (1 portion of your 2 fruit a day), 1–2 tbsp nuts and seeds (protein).

Your lunch plate

A great big tasty salad with rocket (leafy greens), avocado, peppers, olives (other vegetables), beetroot, grated carrot, 3 oatcakes (wholegrains and root veg) and a palm-sized portion of salmon (protein) drizzled with olive oil and balsamic vinegar dressing (good oils).

OR

Spinach, red pepper and cottage cheese frittata (page 150) served with watercress salad (spinach and parsley in the omelette + watercress salad = leafy greens; peppers and onion = other vegetables; eggs = protein; sweet potato = root veg).

Your dinner plate

Roasted vegetables like sweet potato (root veg), peppers, red onion and courgette (other veg) with steamed broccoli spears (leafy greens) and rosemary, lemon and thyme chicken (page 154) (protein).

of fruit. Imagine sitting down to eat that many oranges – it would take you a while! Water is always one of the the best choices for hydration.

These guidelines also suggest using olive oil for cooking and seasoning (taking care not to burn your oil), and use butter in moderation rather than margarine.

Our sources of protein should predominantly be fish, poultry, eggs, pulses (lentils, beans and chickpeas), nuts and seeds. We should eat less lean red meat, and have processed meats like ham and bacon only occasionally.

Our daily dairy intake should be no more than a small matchbox block of cheese or half a cup of live, unsweetened natural yogurt or a small glass of milk – just one of these, not the lot!

It's not just what you eat, it's the way that you eat it ...

No matter what is on our plate, if we are not sitting down to relax and enjoy our meals, our body is unlikely to be getting the true benefits of the food we are eating. Rushed mealtimes, wolfing down our food and grabbing lunch on the run is as bad for our health as it gets. It's so much harder for the body to absorb nutrients if we eat in a state of fight-or-flight.

The vagus nerve connects our bellies to our brains and forms part of the parasympathetic nervous system – also known as the rest-and-digest system. Although the vagus nerve is not the only nerve in this system, it is the most important.

When we are in constant fight-or-flight we switch off our rest-and-digest mode. Important (but non-essential) operations like digestion, immune function and hormone balance are all put on hold while the body prioritises protecting us from the imminent danger we perceive with a rush of adrenalin into our system.

We need to connect our belly to our brain to get the real benefits and true nourishment from the food we eat.

Here are some ideas that can help you connect your belly to your brain:

- Always sit at a table to eat – your desk doesn't count.
- Do not send emails or check social media while you are eating.
- Turn off the TV. Your primal body responds to everything you see. If you start your day watching the news or celebrity chat shows, you are immediately in a state of high alert – your body is ready to fight or flee and you have lost your belly-to-brain connection.

- Slow down. Set your cutlery down between each mouthful. This will feel ridiculous to start with, but it will definitely make you eat more slowly.
- Taste your food. Not just the first mouthful – savour all the different flavours and textures and really taste what you are eating. Enjoy every mouthful.
- Don't jump up from the table the minute you have finished and rush to do the dishes, read emails or watch *EastEnders*. Give yourself a minute or two to digest the food you have just eaten and let it go down.

Happy food memory

Now we have looked at the basics of what to eat and how to eat it, let's think about our relationship with food. When we're thinking of changing our eating habits, it's always a good idea to look back. Often our relationship with food is formed from a young age and most of us can remember a time when food brought us together with other people, gave us a sense of love and wellbeing, or was a source of comfort. Reconnecting with that feeling can bring us more in touch with how food affects our feelings and emotions as well as our physical health.

What is your happy food memory?

Here are some of mine:

- Picking peas with my granda in his vegetable garden and eating them straight from the pod.
- Making soda scones with my granny and eating them hot off the griddle.
- Baking cakes – and licking the spoon – with my mum.

For most of us, food is a way of making social connections with others. What you eat and your attitude to the food on your plate will undoubtedly have an impact on other people. Whether you are single or cooking for a family of six, the food you eat, and more importantly, your attitude to it, will influence others. We are also making food memories for other people. The obvious example here is parents influencing their children (and often older children influencing the rest of the family), but work colleagues, friends enticing us to order an extra dessert, or even the food we notice in someone else's shopping basket can all affect our food choices.

Your food diary

One of the best ways to start to change your diet for the good of your health is to keep a food diary. Keep a note of everything you eat and drink over the next couple of weeks, and when I say everything, I mean everything – the good, the bad and the ugly! Keeping a food diary is a great way to get a clear focus on how you are fuelling your body. No matter whether you are already eating a varied and nutritious diet, or are just starting to think about following a healthier lifestyle, keeping a food diary is a useful exercise to help you make some positive changes.

Week 1 – what do you eat?
Here is a real-life example of a food diary.

	Breakfast	Morning snack	Lunch	Afternoon snack	Dinner	Evening snack
Mon	porridge with honey and nuts	grapes	soup and wheaten bread	chocolate bar and coffee	leftover roast chicken dinner	apple
Tues	toast and peanut butter	scone and coffee (in a meeting!)	chicken wrap	cereal bar and coffee	chilli con carne	banana
Wed	nothing	banana	soup and a sandwich	crisps	chilli con carne with tortilla wrap and salad	chocolate bar
Thurs	porridge with banana	biscuit and tea	chicken wrap	chocolate and coffee	chicken and broccoli pasta bake	glass of wine
Fri	porridge with banana	low-fat yogurt	baked potato and tuna	chocolate and coffee	Indian takeaway	glass of wine and crisps
Sat	scrambled eggs and bacon on toast	pancake and coffee	couscous salad and chicken		steak and chips with salad	glass of wine and crisps
Sun	Weetabix and milk		roast dinner, apple crumble and ice cream		soup and wheaten bread	glass of wine and crisps

The diary opposite is only an example – you should write down exactly what *you* normally eat and don't change anything for the first week. Instead just observe. Use this first week as your 'control' in your own personal food experiment. You will find it useful to refer to after a few weeks, so fill it in as honestly as you can. It is for your eyes only! It is also useful to use your food diary as a check in to see how far you have progressed and celebrate the changes you have made after a couple of weeks.

I always begin work with new clients by asking them to complete a seven-day food diary and they are often shocked by what they are really eating. For instance, take a look at the example on the left – a fairly typical diet. This person, let's call her Sarah, does well with porridge for breakfast, gets her five a day most days, has some oily fish in her diet, eats green, leafy vegetables and does her best to make healthy food that the whole family will enjoy for midweek dinners. Pretty good, I'd say. Look at it more closely, though, and you will notice that she is looking for a snack mid-morning, so may not be eating enough at breakfast. It also looks like she tries hard to make healthy choices at lunchtime, but could do with increasing her vegetable intake here a little. Then notice the obvious dip in the afternoon when she seeks out a chocolate bar and coffee for an energy hit. It looks like she works hard to eat fairly healthy main meals, but her snacks let her down a bit.

Even if you get this nutrition thing and are happy with your diet, give the food diary a go. It might just surprise you.

My approach to a food diary might be a little different to what you are expecting: instead of looking for what is missing, I always look at the good stuff first. Of course all of us can make changes to eat a little better, but all of us have healthy habits too. Look at your diary and pick out three things that you are happy about. For example, Sarah would be able to say:

1. I almost always eat breakfast and make it a healthy choice.

Honey

Honey has been used as part of our 'first-aid' cupboard for generations. Manuka honey is renowned for its antimicrobial properties and has been used in hospitals for wound healing. Honey contains trace minerals, making it a more nutritious choice than sugar, but it's still a relatively high-GI food, so use in moderation.

Superfoods

2.   I aim to get my five portions of fruit and vegetables every day.
3.   I cook healthy meals in bulk to save time and effort.

Let's do a quick check on your diet:

- Do you eat breakfast?
- … and is it (usually) a well-balanced, healthy breakfast?
- Is your diet packed with plants? Vegetables, nuts, fruit, wholegrains and pulses form the basis of the world's healthiest diets.
- Do you eat green, leafy vegetables (e.g. kale, cabbage, broccoli, watercress, rocket, spinach, leeks, chard) every day?
- Do you eat oily fish like salmon, mackerel, herring, trout, sardines or anchovies at least twice a week?
- Do you eat nuts and seeds most days?
- Do you eat brassicas like broccoli, cabbage, cauliflower, Brussels sprouts, kale, pak choi or purple sprouting every day?
- Do you eat some organic food?
- Do you mainly eat food that is in season?
- Do you eat eggs?
- Do you sit at a table to eat all your meals?
- Do you chew your food well?
- Do you drink at least 1.5 litres of water every day?
- Do you avoid sugary foods most of the time?
- Do you cook most of your own food?
- Do you cook with coconut oil?
- Do you use butter instead of margarine?
- Do you use olive oil for dressings and drizzles?
- Do you drink green tea or herbal teas?

If you are able to answer yes to most of these questions, then you are well on your way to eating a diet packed with optimum nutrition. If there are a few nos, then use these questions as inspiration to make some changes to your food diary.

No matter how much you think you need to improve your diet, I'll bet you are already enjoying some foods that are good for you. For example:

- If you like bananas, you are eating some fibre and getting at least one portion of fruit into your diet.
- If you enjoy chilli, you are eating a meal packed with antioxidants (from the tomatoes, onion and vegetables), soluble fibre (from the red kidney beans and vegetables) and protein (from the meat).
- If you drink red wine (in moderation of course), it could be contributing to your antioxidant intake.

Week 2 – what can you change?

In week two, it is time to take some action. Rather than clearing your cupboards of everything you usually eat and having a shopping spree at your local health food shop, think of three small things you could change this week. Keep it simple. Make changes that you are going to enjoy, and always focus on the positives.

Instead of giving yourself a good telling off for what you are not doing, what you shouldn't be eating, or the amount of food you are munching, think about what you could do over the next week to nourish yourself; changes you could make that would make you feel really good about the food on your plate.

For example, this week you could plan to:

1. Eat oily fish twice – maybe salmon for tea on Tuesday and mackerel with tomato and herb salad for lunch on Thursday.
2. Set a 750ml water bottle on your desk and drink it all by the end of the working day.
3. Eat lunch outside at least once.
4. Find a healthy new recipe to add variety to your usual evening meals.
5. Make a healthy lunch for Monday and Tuesday on Sunday evening.
6. Sit at a table to eat all your meals.

Often when we make changes to our diets we focus on cutting things out. Let's look at it another way – choose a food that is good for you and that you enjoy eating and plan to eat more of it this week. Take some time to set yourself some goals for the coming week – what are you going to eat more of? And, just for good measure, what are you going to eat less of?

Week 3 – are you eating enough?

Often when we start to think about making changes to our diet the aim of the game is to cut back. Eat less sugar, smaller portion sizes, reduce our fat intake. What if we turned that around and I asked you to focus on eating more?

Looking at the sample food diary from week one, it seems as though Sarah tries hard to eat a healthy breakfast, lunch and dinner. But notice her desire to snack mid-morning, mid-afternoon and in the evening. The question I would ask is whether she is eating enough at main meals. If not, this could be why she feels so hungry in between. I often find that people eat a very light meal at breakfast and/or lunchtime, leaving them looking for snack foods (which are often unhealthy) between meals.

Although most people think that carbohydrate-rich foods like bread, pasta, rice and potatoes are what keep us feeling fuller for longer, it is usually protein and fat that satiate us better.

Focus on including a palm-sized portion of protein with every meal; include a source of fibre and some good fats too and you are likely to find your temptation to snack is kept in check.

For example:

At breakfast
- add 1–2 tablespoonfuls of nuts and seeds to porridge.
- eat a couple of eggs with toasted rye bread.

At lunchtime
- remember that lunch is a main meal and should not be a snack.
- eat a palm-sized portion of fish or

Superfoods

Mushrooms

The humble chestnut and white mushroom can have as many benefits for our health as their more exotic cousins, like the shiitake, reishi and oyster. Renowned for their immune-boosting properties, mushrooms will take up and absorb whatever they are grown in, including heavy metals and pollutants, so organic are the healthiest choice.

How to store and cook:

- Storing mushrooms on your windowsill to expose them to UV light will increase their vitamin D content.
- Grilled mushrooms maintain more of their antioxidant content than fried mushrooms.

chicken with your salad and swap from bread to seeded oatcakes.

- choose lentil-based soups for additional protein and fibre, and have a side salad and some wheaten bread too so that you max out on veggies and get some extra fibre.

At dinner
- make sure half your plate is packed with vegetables, add a protein source and change your regular potatoes to sweet potatoes for added antioxidants and fibre.
- be creative with vegetables to bump up your fibre intake – add grated carrot, finely sliced leeks or some frozen peas to chilli, curry and stews.

Pomegranates

It seems that pomegranates may contain even more antioxidants than red wine and green tea. Found to offer support for high blood pressure, high cholesterol, oxidative stress, hyperglycaemia and inflammatory conditions, the active polyphenols in pomegranates have even been found to have potential anticarcinogenic effects, and are now widely available.

Superfoods

On the subject of eating more, there are certain foods that we know have extra-special super powers in terms of their nutritional value. Aim to maximise your intake of these foods this week. Eat more:

- green, leafy vegetables
- berries
- oily fish
- wholegrains like oats, buckwheat and quinoa
- nuts and seeds
- yellow and orange fruit and vegetables (e.g. carrots, sweet potato, cantaloupe melon, apricots, butternut squash, etc.)
- herbs and spices like turmeric, rosemary, ginger, garlic, cinnamon, etc.

Week 4 – max up your good fats

Most of us are at least a little bit cautious about eating too much fat, even though we recognise that some fat is good, essential even, for our health and wellbeing. The messages that we receive are so confusing that it's worth delving a bit deeper to discover how to strike a healthy fat balance.

- Eat oily fish at least twice a week. If you can't face the thought of eating oily fish, then consider taking a fish oil supplement containing the essential EPA and DHA fatty acids (page 139).
- Eat a tablespoonful of seeds every day. Try chia, flaxseed, pumpkin, sunflower and sesame seeds. Pop a portion on porridge or cereal, stir into yogurt or sprinkle on to salads.
- Use cold-pressed, organic, extra-virgin olive oil for dressings and drizzles, but don't cook with it at high temperatures as the delicate fatty acids are liable to be damaged.
- Add avocado to your diet. Spread on toasted rye bread for a quick and healthy breakfast, slice into salad at lunch, or mash with some natural yogurt for a healthy dip or snack.
- Eat more houmous. If you buy a ready-made version, make sure it contains olive oil and tahini.
- Use coconut oil for cooking at higher temperatures.
- Switch to butter instead of margarine and use in moderation.
- Eat fewer chips, crisps and fried foods.
- Avoid sunflower oil, margarines and vegetable oils.

This four-week plan is a good foundation to help you make some healthy, positive changes to your diet and get you thinking about the foods you are eating and the impact they are having on your health and wellbeing. As a positive side effect you might notice your energy levels starting to improve, your skin is clearer or your waistline is a little more svelte. Remember, the idea is to make changes to your diet that you enjoy and that you can maintain, rather than a quick-fix diet plan. Once you have the foundations right, I have plenty of ideas for you to explore, including how food can help you sleep well, simple ways to manage sugar cravings or eating for digestive health.

Chapter Two

What's On Your Plate?

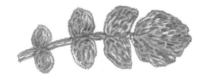

Eat real food!

Healthy eating should never be brown, bland or boring. Neither should it be expensive, made up of ingredients you have never heard of (never mind tasted!), or be so out there that no one else in your family will eat it, leaving you making different dinners for everyone. When it comes to healthy eating, my philosophy is eat real food.

> 'Never go out without a list – a bit basic, but it works!' – EB

Vital shopping tips

The key to eating a healthy diet is having healthy food in your fridge and cupboards, so let's start with how you shop.

- Check out your local greengrocer, butcher, fishmonger or farmers' market and celebrate local produce. Eating local foods that are in season means your plate is packed with optimum nutrition and your food travels fewer miles.
- Never shop when you are hungry. You know this one, right? The days when you are rushing home from work feeling exhausted and ravenous, fly into

the shops and then end up spending a fortune on ready meals and processed food instead of healthy, nourishing food.

- Make a list. Supermarkets in particular are very clever at tempting us to buy stuff we don't need, won't use, or probably don't even like. When was the last time you saw a BOGOF offer on broccoli or berries?
- Take a look in your fridge and cupboards before you pop to the shops so you don't end up with six cans of chickpeas and eight red peppers (although that sounds like the basis of a great soup!). Have a look at what you already have and plan your meals around the food that is there.

Tonight's dinner	Tomorrow's lunch
spinach, red pepper and cottage cheese frittata (page 150) with steamed greens	leftover frittata with avocado and rocket salad
roasted Mediterranean vegetables with grilled halloumi	wholemeal pitta with leftover roasted vegetables, houmous and feta
roast chicken dinner	leftover chicken with Waldorf salad (page 148)

- Plan ahead and meal match. In other words, if you are planning to make bolognese think about making another meal that uses similar ingredients – perhaps a healthy chilli – so that you are saving both on the ingredients and on preparation time. Or think about making more than you need for one meal so you can have leftovers tomorrow.
- Keep your wits about you when you are looking at prices, and look at the small print. Underneath the actual price of the item, you will find the price per kg or 100g in smaller writing. This is useful for comparing like for like, and will mean that you don't pay more for smaller quantities of foods that have been packaged to look like a better deal.
- It is often cheaper to buy loose items rather than pre-packed items – and always check out the offers on the fish and meat counters. This is also a good idea if you are shopping for one or two as you can buy what you need rather than too much, meaning less food waste and a cheaper shop.

- Choose something different every week. If you usually buy broccoli, pop a cauliflower in your trolley; if you always eat apples, try pears for a change. Not only will you get more variety in your diet, but more nutrition too.

> 'I find the best way to manage costs and to save time is to plan ahead. I decide on several dishes and then do a weekly cook-off.' – LT

- Buy real food. If a food has to tell you it contains natural ingredients, is low fat, fortified with vitamins and minerals, or any other such sales pitch, think twice. Healthy food rarely has to make a song and dance about the benefits it offers. Fill your basket with food that is as close to nature as possible and you can't go too far wrong.

What to choose, what to avoid

- Always pick up a variety of fruit and vegetables. The more variety the better, so I suggest especially that you throw in plenty of colourful vegetables and think about getting as many different types of fruit and veg into your basket as possible. Always include green, leafy vegetables as well (they are your nutritional powerhouses), some brassicas (cabbage, kale, pak choi, broccoli, Brussels sprouts) and a few alliums (onions, garlic, leeks, scallions, shallots). In the fruit section, look out for fruit that grows locally. Don't overstock, though, as this stuff will go off quickly and end up as expensive compost – shop little and often for fruit and vegetables.
- Don't forget about fish. Pick up some oily varieties like mackerel, herring, trout, salmon or sardines, remembering to look out for the little Marine Stewardship Council (MSC) flag that tells you it is sustainable. Swordfish, shark, tuna and marlin tend to contain higher than average levels of mercury, so are best kept to a minimum. Tinned fish is ideal for packed lunches – sardines, mackerel and pilchards are richer in the essential omega-3 fats than tuna and they are less likely to be contaminated by pollutants and mercury as these fish are lower down the food chain.
- When it comes to the butcher, remember that red meat should be eaten in moderation – in this case, moderation means no more than twice a week.

What's in season?

Know what's in season. Most of us have lost a real connection with the food we eat. We eat strawberries at Christmas and tomatoes in January, forgetting that Mother Nature has a fine balance of seasons. When we are in tune with the seasons we want comforting foods in winter when we should be hibernating and fresh, crisp salads in spring and summer when we feel lighter and more energetic.

Spring

As we shed our winter layers and the days get longer and brighter, our appetites turn to clean greens and lighter foods.

What's in season?

- cabbage
- cauliflower
- celeriac
- grapefruit
- leeks
- onions
- oranges
- pak choi
- parsnip
- peppers
- pomegranate
- purple-sprouting broccoli
- rhubarb
- scallions
- sweet potato
- turnip

Summer

The living is easy. Spend less time in the kitchen and more time eating outside. Enjoy the best of the season –fresh, crisp salads and seasonal, juicy fruit.

What's in season?

- asparagus
- aubergines
- beetroots
- blackcurrants
- broad beans
- broccoli
- cabbage
- carrots
- cavolo nero
- courgettes
- fennel
- globe artichokes
- gooseberries
- lettuce
- nectarines
- new potatoes
- onions
- pak choi
- peas
- peppers
- radishes
- runner beans
- sorrel
- spinach
- tomatoes
- watercress

Autumn

The season of abundance when we harvest and store the food we have grown over the summer to feed us through the winter.

What's in season?

- apples
- aubergines
- beetroots
- blackberries
- broccoli
- Brussels sprouts
- cabbage
- carrots
- cavolo nero
- celeriac
- celery
- kale
- kohlrabi
- leeks
- lettuce
- onions
- pak choi
- parsnip
- pears
- peas
- peppers
- plums
- pomegranate
- pumpkin
- sweet potato
- Swiss chard
- turnip

Winter

Winter is made for snuggling up and hibernating. We want foods to comfort, nourish and warm us.

What's in season?

- apples
- beetroots
- Bramley apples
- Brussels sprouts
- cabbage
- cauliflower
- celeriac
- celery
- chicory
- clementines
- grapefruit
- Jerusalem artichoke
- kale
- leeks
- onions
- oranges
- pak choi
- parsnip
- pears
- pomegranate
- rhubarb
- swede
- sweet potato
- turnip

Good choices are some minced steak to make chilli or bolognese (organic is best), or a leg of Irish lamb for Sunday roast, with leftovers for a stir-fry next week. Chicken should not be cheap. If it is, it may not be the best nutritional choice. I would recommend buying organic chicken, which can be more expensive, so buy the whole chicken or look out for chicken thighs or legs instead of the more expensive organic breasts. They are delicious cooked with a marinade, or used as the base for a chicken stew – try cooking them with tinned tomatoes, some root vegetables, onions, leeks, herbs and a can of butter beans to make your meat go further.

- Cured and smoked meats like bacon, ham and sausages should be avoided, or at least eaten very infrequently.
- It's easy to be tempted by shiny labels and nutritional claims in the dairy aisle if you are not careful. Stay away from anything that says low fat, reduced fat, low calorie, or that makes any claims about weight. Research now tells us that a moderate intake of full-fat milk may be preferable to skimmed milk for weight management. This could be thanks to fat making us feel more satiated, or the fact that these foods tend to contain less sugar. Unfortunately that does not give us a licence to start guzzling cream with every meal, but just a reminder that it may be preferable to replace some of our low-fat options with full-fat alternatives. Some dairy products tend to be more nutritious than others. Full-fat natural yogurt that says 'bio' or 'live' on the label and cottage cheese (which is a natural probiotic food) are good options to help keep your good gut bacteria happy. Next is the butter v. margarine debate. Put it like this: would you rather eat a food that is natural or a food that is processed? Butter it is, and organic if you can get it – pesticide residues are fat-soluble, which makes

Superfoods

Black pepper

Although we use only small amounts, black pepper has important health benefits thanks to its antioxidant, antimicrobial, antidepressant and gastro-protective ingredients.

Black pepper seems to have fat-burning properties and is found in nutritional supplements designed for weight loss. It is also thought to improve the bioavailability of curcumin from turmeric, so add a grind of black pepper any time you're using turmeric.

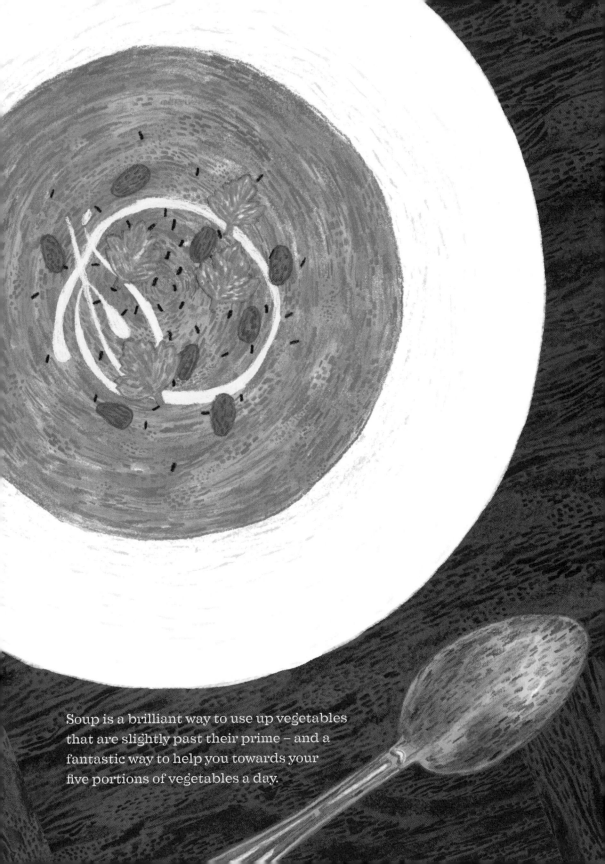

Soup is a brilliant way to use up vegetables that are slightly past their prime – and a fantastic way to help you towards your five portions of vegetables a day.

Celery

This humble vegetable contains more than its fair share of flavonoids like zeaxanthin, lutein and betacarotene, which have been linked to improved eyesight, immune support, anticancer effects, lowering inflammation and reducing heart disease risk.

organic the best choice. How about some cheese? Cottage, goat's or feta are all good choices. Some people find that goat's and sheep's cheeses, like feta, tend to be easier to digest than cheese made with cow's milk. Look out for unpasteurised or raw cheeses too as these can benefit your healthy gut bugs in the same way as yogurt. If you want a dairy alternative to milk, give soya a wide berth and try coconut or almond milk instead, unsweetened of course. Although soya milk and soya yogurt are often thought of as healthy alternatives, these unfermented forms of soya can be difficult to digest, and may interfere with thyroid function and upset female hormone balance. If you want to add soya into your diet, then look out for fermented foods like tofu, miso or tempeh.

- Bread is no longer the regional food it originally was. The ingredients of a loaf of bread used to be flour, yeast, water. These days, the bread we buy typically contains wheat flour (with added calcium, iron, niacin and thiamin), water, yeast, soya flour, emulsifiers (E471, E472e), preservative E282 and flour treatment agent (ascorbic acid).
  - » E471 is manufactured from glycerine and fatty acids which are normally obtained from hydrogenated soya bean oil. It's used as an 'anti-staling' agent so your bread lasts longer.
  - » E472e – esters of synthetic fats – is produced from glycerol, natural fatty acids and another organic acid (acetic, lactic, tartaric, citric). It is used to strengthen the dough to give a springy, chewy texture.
  - » E282 is used as a mould inhibitor and is thought to be linked to migraine headaches.

When choosing bread, why not think of it it as a treat, spending a little more to get better quality or making your own using good-quality ingredients. Sourdough bread from a local bakery (or home-made) is ideal, but if you can't get this, then try rye bread or unsweetened wheaten bread as low-GI alternatives.

- Carefully chosen canned foods can be some of your healthiest store cupboard essentials. Tinned tomatoes and passata tend to be cheaper and healthier than pasta sauces. Canned beans and chickpeas make a handy and healthy protein choice and are a great way of adding bulk to casseroles, curries, chillis and stews. Lentils are a good choice too – look out for different varieties. I tend to choose red lentils for soups, puy lentils to bulk out bolognese and green lentils as the base for a salad. While you are in this section, don't forget to pick up those couple of tins of fish, like sardines or mackerel, for lunches.
- Choose plenty of olives, capers, sun-dried tomatoes and artichokes. This aisle is a treasure trove of ingredients packed with phytochemicals and health-giving properties that will add a taste of the Mediterranean to your everyday meals.
- Nuts, seeds and nut butter are packed with nutrition and can make a healthful addition to breakfast, salads, snacks and stir-fries. Keep an eye on the cost per kg as nuts vary greatly in price. Of course, the healthy options are the unroasted, unsalted nuts and seeds. Also look out for sugar-free nut

Onions

If onions make you cry, it is thanks to their allyl sulphide content, the same stuff that has been credited with their ability to help balance blood-sugar levels and prevent hypoglycaemia.

Onions are also an important source of the antioxidant quercetin, which has powerful anti-inflammatory and antihistamine effects. This everyday vegetable also has a big impact on our gut microbiome thanks to its inulin content. Inulin is a prebiotic fibre that is indigestible to us, but that our good bacteria thrive on.

Although onions are good for us whether we eat them raw or cooked, it seems that we get more of the sulphur-containing compounds if we can eat them raw. If you find the taste too strong, try chives, scallions or red onions instead of white onions.

Superfoods

butters. Do your bit for the planet and take care to avoid nut butter with palm oil, though.

- Herbs and spices – even dried ones – are full of powerful nutrients. My favourites are turmeric, cinnamon, cayenne and paprika, and I use sea salt and black pepper every day. Asian supermarkets can offer great value on fresh and dried herbs and spices.

- Don't bypass frozen foods as there are some healthy gems to be found. Frozen vegetables like peas, broad beans and spinach are great for maximising nutrition in lots of different dishes, and the variety in frozen vegetables available now can save you time, money and effort in the kitchen. In the same way, if you are eating berries every day, check out the frozen

Coffee

You may be surprised to see coffee included as a superfood as it often gets a bad press thanks to its stimulant effects and links with raised blood pressure. Some people are genetically more sensitive to caffeine than others, so coffee should not be on everyone's list of superfoods, but good quality coffee (i.e. not the instant stuff) contains phytochemical and antioxidants thought to exert potential health benefits, including:

- improved mood and energy levels (thanks to its stimulant effects)
- fat-burning properties as it increases our basal metabolic rate

- enhanced physical performance
- protective effects on the liver
- potential benefits for prevention of dementia and Parkinson's
- reduced risk of type 2 diabetes
- improved memory and cognitive function

But avoid coffee if you have high blood pressure, anxiety or a tendency towards diarrhoea.

Of course, it is the quality of coffee that matters. As coffee is one of the most mass-produced crops in the world it tends to be heavily sprayed with pesticides and fungicides. When buying your coffee, make sure you are sourcing a fair-trade, organic product, and choose ground coffee or coffee beans rather than instant.

ones and keep fresh berries as a seasonal treat. Frozen fish can also be a handy standby for weeknight meals, as long as you choose the plain varieties, not the breaded or battered options.

- Take particular care when you are choosing your breakfast cereal. Beware of claims like low fat, lighter, fortified with vitamins and minerals, etc. – these claims are often no more than a ploy to get us to buy high-sugar, highly processed junk food for breakfast. Jumbo porridge oats are safe enough (just not the flavoured varieties), and if you hunt carefully, you will be able to find low-sugar granola and muesli. Just remember that 5g per 100g or less is low sugar, so keep that in mind when checking labels.
- Although the biscuit aisle tends to be a recipe for disaster, pop a pack of oatcakes into your trolley to have with lunches or with a little nut butter as a healthy snack.
- When it comes to coffee, why not try some fair-trade, organic, ground coffee instead of instant, so coffee becomes a treat, rather than something you drink all day in a processed form. Green and herbal teas make a refreshing and healthy change from black tea. Look out for teas based on lavender and lemon balm which are particularly calming, or peppermint and fennel to support your digestive system. Caffeinated drinks like tea, coffee and green tea are fine in moderation, but some people are particularly sensitive to caffeine and may be better off drinking herbal teas instead. Decaf tea and coffee tends to be decaffeinated using solvents which may have detrimental health effects.
- Eggs are packed full of nutrition as well as being economical and so versatile – I think that they are an essential part of any healthy shopping basket. By preference, I would choose organic free-range every time.

Deciphering food labels

Looking at food labels can be confusing at the best of times, but you don't need a food science degree to work out what's in your food if you follow some basic rules.

Most foods include a nutrition panel on the back of the pack detailing calories, fat content, saturated fats, carbohydrate, sugar, protein and salt per 100g. Sometimes you will also see the amount per portion size in this panel too, and some food manufacturers highlight the nutrition content as a traffic-light system on the front of the pack as a quick reference. Of course the manufacturer is keen for you to buy their food, so this front-of-pack labelling is not always there.

- Be wary of any food making excessive claims and boasts. Phrases such as 'low sugar', 'low fat' and 'fortified with vitamins and minerals' are often trying to dress an unhealthy food up as something more than it is.
- Look closely at the ingredients list. If it reads like something from a science lab, leave the food on the shelf. If you recognise all the ingredients – especially if you might find them in your kitchen cupboards – then you are safe enough.
- Also think about the order in which the ingredients are listed. If sugar is high on the list, think twice about buying that food. Remember that sugar has many guises, so look out for healthy-sounding ingredients like honey, molasses and maple syrup, as well as hydrolysed starch, modified

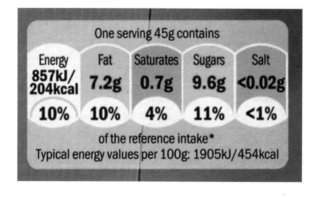

Front of pack labels show amounts as per the manufacturer's recommended portion size.

Nutrition

Typical values	100g contains	40g contains	% RI*	RI* for an average adult
Energy	1550kJ	620kJ		8400kJ
	367kcal	147kcal	7%	2000kcal
Fat	1.9g	0.8g	1%	70g
of which saturates	0.4g	0.2g	1%	20g
Carbohydrate	71.8g	28.7g		
of which sugars	13.9g	5.6g	6%	90g
Fibre	10.8g	4.3g		
Protein	10.1g	4.0g		
Salt	0.6g	0.2g	3%	6g

Pack contains 18 servings
*Reference intake of an average adult (8400kJ / 2000kcal)

These labels, usually found on the back of packets, show nutritional values per 100g and per recommended portion size.

starch, starch, carbohydrate, corn syrup, treacle, fruit syrup and anything ending in -ose (dextrose, glucose, fructose, sucralose, etc.) These ingredients are just sugar by another name.

> 'By shopping online I'm not tempted to overspend on food I don't need or on tempting treats in the aisles.' – PK

- Take a look at the nutritional information and train your eye to check the sugar content before anything else – 5g of sugar per 100g or less is low.

- Ignore the calorie count, as not all calories are created equally. I know that this is a big leap of faith if you have been a lifelong dieter, so let me explain. While it is true that eating a high-calorie diet will have consequences for your waistline, some types of calories are more likely to end up contributing to our bingo wings and muffin tops than others. If the calories you are eating come mainly from sugar and refined carbohydrates, that is a sure-fire way of piling on the pounds. However, if they are from fat and protein, it's likely that food will leave you feeling fuller for longer, help your metabolism and not end up as your spare tyre – calories are complicated. I think a good rule of thumb is to watch your intake of sugar and refined carbohydrates rather than your calorie intake.

- If you want to work out the number of teaspoonfuls of sugar per portion, then divide the number of grams per portion by four. For example, if there are 16g of sugar per portion, that means there are 4 teaspoonfuls in a portion. But remember that most of us eat more than the recommended portion – the small portion sizes recommended can be another trick to make it look as though a food is a healthy choice. A good example is your breakfast cereal. Have you ever measured a 30g portion of cornflakes? It is shockingly tiny. In some of my workshops I ask people to pour out a portion size of cereal and I find that most people weigh out at least twice the manufacturer's recommended amount.

- Not all fats are bad, even the saturated sort. A good example is a bag of Brazil nuts, which lists 68g fat per 100g, with about 7g as saturated fat. If you thought fat was bad, then Brazil nuts would go nowhere near your shopping trolley. However, if you consider that this fat contributes to the normal functioning of your metabolism, improves skin health, helps regulate inflammation, and supports your immune system, you might think differently about Brazil nuts. Of all the fats in our diet, industrially produced trans fats are the worst offenders for our health. These processed fats have been associated with an increased risk of cardiovascular disease and are found in margarine, manufactured cakes, crisps, biscuits, pastries and fried foods in restaurants and takeaways. Although there is no legal requirement to list trans fat content on food labels in the UK, in recent years the food industry has voluntarily reduced the levels of trans fats in the foods they produce.

- Take a look at the listed salt content. We should aim to have no more than 6g per day; anything over 1.5g per 100g means high salt content.
- Pick up a couple of versions of the same food. For example, two different packets of biscuits, two varieties of yogurts or two kinds of cereals and compare the labels. This kind of comparison should help ensure that the healthier version ends up in your trolley.

What about organic?

I advise trying to reduce your pesticide load as much as possible. One of the simplest ways to do this is to choose organic food. The costs of organic have thankfully come down a bit over the last few years, so it's a more viable option.

When shopping, I tend to buy organic meat, chicken, eggs, butter, oils, nuts and seeds. A simple rule of thumb is the higher up the food chain, the more concentrated the pesticide residue load in that food is likely to be. Buy the best-quality meat and chicken you can afford and make it go further by bulking it out with pulses and using leftovers wisely.

'I have recently started to order my meat and fish in bulk. I would rather eat good quality less often.' – JC

When it comes to fruit and vegetables, some tend to be sprayed more than others. In the USA the Environmental Working Group publishes the Clean 15 and Dirty Dozen lists every year. Although this is an American resource and our farming regulations are slightly different, I think this is still a useful guide to help us to reduce our intake of pesticide residues. In general, foods that grow above ground and have a quick growth cycle (e.g. leafy greens, berries) tend to have higher pesticide residues than foods that grow below ground (e.g. root vegetables). Remember that no matter whether you are choosing organic or not, fruit and vegetables are an essential part of a healthy diet. If you can only afford to choose organic for a limited amount of your shopping, then I suggest choosing the organic option if you're buying any of the foods on the Dirty Dozen list.

Clean 15, Dirty Dozen

When buying non-organic produce, choose the foods on the 'Clean 15' list as they have been shown to have the lowest levels of pesticide residue.

Clean 15	Dirty Dozen
sweetcorn	strawberries
avocado	spinach
pineapple	nectarines
cabbage	apples
onion	peaches
peas	pears
papaya	cherries
asparagus	grapes
mango	celery
aubergine	tomatoes
honeydew melon	peppers
kiwi	potatoes
cantaloupe	
cauliflower	
grapefruit	

Affordable organics

If you're thinking of trying organic foods, these ideas should make them a bit easier on your pocket:

- Shop in 'budget' supermarkets where you'll often find organic food at a better price.

- Shop around and source local organic butchers and farmers. Many organic producers sell straight from their farm or at farmers' markets, which can be better value than buying your meat from a supermarket.
- Ask your supplier about recipe ideas for cheaper cuts of organic meat. This means you can still benefit from eating organic at a more affordable price.
- Eat less meat. Meat is the most expensive part of any meal – especially when it is organic. Eating meat less often is not only good for your wallet, but makes sense for your health too. Have at least one meat-free day a week. Use pulses as an alternative protein source.
- Whether you have a garden or just a window box, growing your own vegetables is a sure-fire way to guarantee you are eating organic crops. Start with something easy to grow like rocket or peas and grow the stuff you like to eat. Zero pesticides, zero food miles!
- It is also worth considering an organic vegetable box delivery as this can work out cheaper than buying the same things from the supermarket. It may also encourage you to vary your diet as you tend to get whatever is in season and the contents change each week. Share with friends if there is too much for you to eat in one week, or get a fortnightly delivery.

'How do I eat well but save money at the checkout? Only one word needed to answer this question – soup!' – RM

Tips for eating away from home

I know from my own experience and from talking to clients that eating out can sometimes be a challenge if you want to make nutritious choices. As healthy eating has increasingly become the trendy new thing, lots of cafes, restaurants and convenience stores have at least a few good choices on their shelves and menus if you know what to look for. So whether you are popping into a garage to grab a snack on the road, or eating out, here are a few ideas that might help you to eat well when you're away from home.

At the airport/in the skies

Whether you are travelling for business or pleasure, making healthy food choices will mean you arrive at your destination feeling refreshed and energised.

- If you are on a red-eye flight, first thing in the morning, your body will thank you for a protein-rich breakfast. Most airports serve porridge these days and if you add some nuts, seeds and fruit, it is an option that will set you up well for the day. If you prefer a cooked breakfast, then go for scrambled eggs or an omelette with tomatoes and mushrooms – and do your best to ignore the croissants and pastries. These are more likely to cause a spike and subsequent crash in your blood sugar levels, leaving you grumpy, tired and wanting more sugar and carbs later in the day.
- If you reach the airport at lunch or dinner time, stick to the principle of choosing a protein-based food like chicken, houmous, beans or fish and having plenty of vegetables or salad with it, and you can't go too far wrong.
- Right beside the chocolate and crisps in the airport shop you can always find a healthy snack bar (which although not the best choice ever, is likely to be better than a bar of chocolate – look for one containing nuts and seeds, and check the sugar content), some nuts and seeds or dried fruit if you get the munchies.
- Keep well hydrated. Take a bottle of water on the flight with you and sip it regularly throughout your journey. Drink herbal teas instead of coffee at the airport and avoid the temptation of alcohol – at least until you reach your destination.

- Digestion is affected by flying, so while on board go for light options like soups, salads, natural yogurt and peppermint tea to reduce gas, wind and bloating.
- Tomato juice is the quintessential airline drink and makes a great choice as it is easy to digest and packed with nutrition. Interestingly, it is thought that our sense of taste can be influenced by other senses, so the high decibel level in the airline cabin means our palate registers sweet tastes less intensely, while the taste known as umami is heightened. This could explain the popularity of tomato juice on aeroplanes.
- All airlines now serve healthy options. Seed and nut bars, porridge, olives, meze snack boxes, couscous and noodle pots are better choices than crisps, croque-monsieurs or sweets.

On the road

If you find yourself at the motorway sevices or petrol station looking for a healthy bite to eat, here are a few ideas to help you out.

- Most convenience stores now have a hot-food counter where you can pick up something handy and nutritious like soup and wheaten bread. Add some protein – like a snack pack of Brazil nuts or almonds or some cooked chicken pieces – and you have a relatively healthy meal.
- Beside the sandwiches you will find salad boxes. Choose one with egg, chicken or tuna as these tend to be lower in salt than the ham or cheese versions.
- Look out for protein pots in the fresh-food section. Often a combination of spinach with a boiled egg, or houmous and carrot sticks, these healthy snacks will help maintain your concentration for driving and provide a more sustainable source of energy than a quick fix of crisps or chocolate.
- If you like to nibble when driving, choose packs of dried fruit and nuts, or take some grapes to munch on, which are at least a better choice than sweets or chocolate.
- If you need a sweet treat, look out for protein bars like Kind, Bounce or Nakd bars as an occasional snack as they will keep you going much longer than any other sweet treat.

Eating out

I think eating out is one of life's great pleasures and sometimes we should just eat for pleasure rather than because it is good for us! If you are out and want to choose healthier options, then there are a few basic principles I would suggest.

- Bypass the bread basket. If you want a little morsel to whet your appetite, lots of restaurants serve olives and nuts that will do the trick.
- Stick to starter and main course and skip dessert to keep your sugar levels in check.
- For starter, choose something like a crab or prawn salad or soup, or try the vegetarian option, which will help to increase your veggie intake.
- For main course, think protein! Have a look at the menu and you will find a few protein options to choose from. Steak, fish, chicken or bean-based vegetarian dishes are ideal. Add a vegetable side like steamed greens, house salad or seasonal vegetables and share the side of carbohydrate-based foods – perhaps baby boiled potatoes or some rice.
- Italian menus are heavy on pasta and pizza, but start with a tomato and mozzarella salad to get your protein quota, and if you love pizza, choose a thin-based one with a vegetable topping served with a great big salad.
- If Indian food is your thing, then check out the tandoori options as they are marinated in spices and baked in a tandoor oven and usually served with a vegetable curry. Lentil and chickpea dishes are good options too, and choose tomato-based sauces rather than the creamy ones. Instead of doubling up on the carbohydrates with naan and rice, go halves with your dining partner. Order a vegetable side dish like sag paneer or chana dhal instead of extra rice.
- The takeaway food scene is changing. Although many Chinese and Asian takeaway meals are laden with sugary sauces and deep-fried foods, there are now some great healthier options – such as sides of brown rice and steamed greens – so look around for these alternatives. Look for coconut-based curries, fish-based dishes, steamed vegetables, and order a side of Asian slaw if it's on the menu.

Chapter Three

Sugar Fix

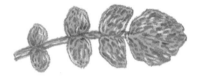

Pure, white and deadly sound like adjectives to describe a class A drug, but the same words have been used to describe sugar. However, we don't have to buy it undercover – sugar is available in every corner shop and supermarket and we can't get enough of it. We love sugar in all its forms. Even some of the vegetables and fruit we buy have been modified to maximise their natural sweetness so that they appeal to our palates.

Although sugar has only hit the headlines fairly recently, nutritionists have known about its detrimental effects on our health for years. Most of us consume more than is good for us with dire consequences for our long-term health. Over time, a high-sugar diet makes our cells resistant to the effects of insulin, and it is this phenomenon that is at the crux of sugar's ill effects on our health and wellbeing. Insulin resistance increases risk of serious health problems like type 2 diabetes, coronary heart disease, obesity, inflammatory conditions and cancer.

While a little bit of sugar every now and then is unlikely to cause much harm, it is the vast quantities of the stuff we consume

'When I gave up refined sugar I was amazed at the results. My friends noticed how much brighter my skin was, I had much more energy, felt healthy and began to really enjoy the taste of food again.' – NG

that is the problem. I don't think we need to totally eliminate sugar from our diet, but I do think we need to take steps to seriously curb our sugar intake.

I find that when clients at my clinic cut back on the amount of sugar they eat, they notice almost immediate benefits. Improved energy, better mood, fewer cravings and weight loss are the most common benefits after just a few weeks off the white stuff.

Once we get our sweet tooth under control I think there is room in most people's diet for the occasional sweet treat.

'Now that I am sugar free it's very hard to believe that I used to be the way I was – when I look back, I am really shocked by the way sugar controlled my life. Now my mind is clear and focused, my skin feels healthy and I am relaxed and rational – a totally different person.' – JS

As a self-confessed chocaholic, I know first-hand how hard it can be to give up sugar, but I firmly believe that the benefits of cutting back far outweigh the cravings.

Sugar on the brain ...

Take one little bite of a chocolate bar and it is an instant love affair. The taste receptors on our tongues send a spark to our brains that something good is going to happen. Our brains' reward centres are then activated to release a surge of dopamine and serotonin, so we feel the sugar love.

This is lovely if we only eat sugary stuff every now and then, but when we gorge on too much, too often, things start to get a bit out of control and we end up addicted. Too much of a good thing and our brains' reward centres start to become overactivated. We get bursts of dopamine and surges of serotonin, leaving us craving more sugar and depleted of these two feel-good neurotransmitters until we end up crashing with exhaustion and low mood.

Insulin resistance

When we overindulge in sugar and bombard our little cells with too much sweet stuff we end up in a state of insulin resistance – our cells stop listening to the insulin signal, so our pancreas releases more insulin in a vain attempt to get our blood sugar under control. Over time, the pancreas can no longer produce such high levels of insulin and our blood sugar levels increase to a consistently high level as a result, increasing risk of type 2 diabetes.

The signs of insulin resistance include lethargy, hunger, poor concentration, weight gain around the middle, high blood pressure and high cholesterol. They do not show themselves at first but develop over time. Insulin resistance can be successfully managed through dietary changes and a targeted exercise plan.

Stop the sugar cycle

There is a way to crack the sugar cycle – it just takes a few adjustments and some focus on our diet.

Step 1: Know the enemy

Before we can cut back on sugar, we need to find out where it is lurking.

Understanding food labels

Food labels give us lots of useful information about how much sugar is in our food.

- Take a look at the ingredients list. Ingredients are listed in descending order of weight. If sugar is near the top of the list, you are probably looking at a high-sugar food.
- Look out for any ingredient ending in -ose (e.g. sucrose, dextrose, lactose, fructose, maltose). They are all forms of the same thing – sugar. Syrups such as corn and rice, as well as honey, agave and molasses are sugar in disguise too.
- Look at the nutritional information to check the amount of sugar per 100g. Anything less than 5g per 100g is low and more than 22.5g per 100g is high.

To help you visualise how much sugar is in your food remember that 4g is the equivalent to 1 teaspoonful, so check the nutrition panel to see how many grams are in one portion and divide by 4 to work out how many teaspoonfuls are in each portion.

Coconut

Coconut has made its way into our diets in a big way in recent years, with coconut milk and coconut oil becoming particularly popular. Rich in fibre, vitamins C, E, B1, B3, B5 and B6 as well as a good source of iron, potassium, selenium, calcium and magnesium, there is good reason why we can't get enough of the stuff. Although coconut is high in saturated fats, these are medium-chain fatty acids (MCFAs) which have particular health consequences. MCFAs are metabolised easily and effectively by the liver, which means that instead of posing a risk to heart health they seem to have potential benefits instead. Linked with reduced risk of high blood pressure, reduced LDL (low-density lipoprotein) cholesterol, potential benefits for reducing risk of obesity and insulin resistance, coconut oil seems like an important ingredient in our health arsenal.

A key ingredient in coconut is lauric acid. With its antibacterial, antifungal effects, lauric acid can help support healthy gut flora and protect us against infection.

Coconut water is a great recovery drink after exercise as it is packed with electrolytes to replenish lost salts. Coconut oil has a relatively high smoke point in comparison with other plant-based oils, making it one of the safest oils to cook with.

How to use:
- In cooking – as it is stable even at high temperatures.
- Add a spoonful of coconut oil to good quality coffee and froth it up to make a healthy and tasty drink thought to have fat-burning properties.
- Drink coconut water for post-exercise recovery.
- Snack on flaked coconut to satisfy sweet cravings and balance blood sugar.
- Try coconut yogurt as a dairy-free snack.
- Use coconut milk as a base ingredient for curry. Choose the full-fat version to get the health benefits.

Superfoods

Hidden sugar

Sometimes hidden sugar can catch us out. Even some of our favourite savoury foods can be high in sugar, and low-fat foods are often packed full of sugar to make them tasty.

- Take a look at the nutritional information panel on your favourite carton of soup or jar of bolognese sauce – its sugar content might surprise you.
- Fruit contains more sugar than vegetables. Keep an eye on your fruit intake and don't eat more than two portions in one day, remembering that fruit that grows locally is usually lower in sugar than tropical varieties.
- Fizzy drinks, cordials, smoothies and fruit juices all contain sugar – if we are drinking a lot of these, we will definitely be taking in more sugar than our bodies can handle.

Check the sugar content of your breakfast cereal. Even wholesome-seeming granola and muesli can be high sugar because of the dried fruit content. I've had a look at some healthy-looking cereals for you to see what's on the label:

	sugar per 100g	sugar content in a recommended portion size
Kellogg's Ancient Legends Spelt Granola	28g	13g
No-Added Sugar Alpen	16g	7.2g
Jordans Natural Muesli	15.8g	7.1g
Special K	15g	4.5g
Lizi's Low Sugar Granola	3.8g	1.9g
Rude Health No Flamin' Raisins Muesli	3.2g	1.9g

Good sugar, bad sugar ...

In truth, sugar is sugar, no matter what way you look at it. Of course sugar that is found naturally in fruit, or the lactose in milk, is a better choice than chocolate bars or fizzy drinks, because at least you are getting the benefits of additional nutrients and fibre or protein, which help to slow the release of sugar.

Hidden sugars come in all forms: fruit sugars, dried fruit, fruit juice, honey, agave syrup, coconut sugar, artificial sweeteners and xylitol are all sugar in one form or another. Although natural sweeteners like these are a better choice than sugar, it all adds up and these foods may contribute to fluctuating blood glucose levels.

Artificial sweeteners like aspartame are not a great alternative as the jury is out on their long-term health effects. The idea behind cutting back on sweet stuff is to retrain our palates so we do not crave sugar so much. If we continue to eat foods that taste sweet, it may make it more difficult to curb cravings.

How much sugar is in your food?
Look at your food diary and highlight any foods that you think may contain sugar. Alternatively you might find it useful to use a food diary app (e.g. MyFitnessPal) to work out your sugar intake each day. Once you identify where sugar is lurking, you can then make an informed decision about what to change. Don't forget that some of the sugar in your diet may be cunningly disguised.

'Writing everything down every day means you can see what you are doing and helps with control.' – GC

As an example, let's take a closer look at a typical day on a 'healthy' diet so that I can show you what I mean about those hidden sugars.

breakfast	no-added-sugar muesli, banana, glass of orange juice
mid-morning snack	pot of low-fat strawberry yogurt coffee with milk
lunch	chicken salad sandwich, half-carton of fresh tomato and basil soup glass of water
afternoon snack	low-fat cereal bar tea with milk
dinner	salmon, pasta, peas, spinach and sweet chilli sauce glass of water

If you add up all the sugar in this menu, you end up with a whopping intake of 122g – almost five times the WHO recommended maximum intake of 25g per day. If the

	Calories kcal	Carbs g	Fat g	Protein g	Sodium mg	Sugar g
Breakfast						
orange juice, 237ml	112	26	0	2	2	21
Jordans – Natural Muesli, 45g inc semi skim	208	33	4	8	0	12
banana, 126g	124	30	0	1	1	19
Total	**444**	**89**	**4**	**11**	**3**	**52**
Lunch						
Tesco – chicken salad sandwich, 1 pack	434	45	14	31	710	5
Tesco – tomato and basil soup, ½ carton (300g)	130	15	5	3	600	13
Total	**564**	**60**	**19**	**34**	**1,310**	**18**
Dinner						
peas, 80g	70	12	1	5	370	4
penne, 1 cup	200	42	1	7	10	2
salmon, 1 fillet, steamed	160	0	4	23	240	0
Sainsbury's – sweet chilli sauce, 1 tbsp	29	7	1	1	76	6
spinach, raw, 1 cup	7	1	0	1	24	0
Total	**466**	**62**	**7**	**37**	**720**	**12**
Snacks						
Yoplait – low-fat yogurt, strawberry, 175g	163	24	3	9	110	24
Nakd – cocoa orange bar, 35g	145	16	7	4	0	14
coffee with milk	22	1	2	0	18	1
tea with milk, 1 large mug (250 ml)	20	1	1	1	0	1
Total	**350**	**42**	**13**	**14**	**128**	**40**
Daily Total	**1,824**	**253**	**43**	**96**	**2,161**	**122**

menu also included a spoonful of sugar in each cup of tea and coffee and a can of fizzy drink, it would bump the sugar intake up by an additional 49g.

Where is all the sugar coming from?

For the purposes of analysis, I am using brands that are fairly typical of their food type in terms of sugar content.

Breakfast: 52g sugar
- This healthy-seeming breakfast provides twice the WHO recommended sugar intake for the day, even before we have left the house.
- This no-added sugar muesli contains dried fruit (a sugar source) – one portion contains 12g of sugar per bowl.
- A medium-sized banana adds an extra 19g to our bowl.
- The glass of orange juice packs 21g of sugar (more than 5 teaspoonfuls!) into just one small glass.

Lunch: 18g sugar
- Soup and a sandwich seems like a sensible choice for lunch, but there are more than 3 teaspoonfuls of sugar (13g) in the half-carton of soup, which makes it look a little less appealing.

Dinner: 12g sugar
- This healthy-sounding dinner is great until we pour on the tablespoonful of sweet chilli sauce, instantly adding 6g of sugar.

Snacks: 40g sugar
- Choosing a flavoured low-fat yogurt adds up to 24g of sugar to our daily intake – six teaspoonfuls.
- Each of these 'healthy' snack bars contains 14g (3.5 teaspoonfuls) of sugar.

Cinnamon

Cinnamon is one of the most commonly used spices in the world and has a place in both sweet and savoury dishes. Many of its health benefits have been attributed to its coumarin content. Cinnamon has antioxidant, anti-inflammatory, anti-diabetic, antimicrobial, lipid-lowering effects and has been reported to act against neurological disorders like Parkinson's and Alzheimer's.

Superfoods

Small changes

Now let's change the menu a little to show how some simple changes can dramatically improve things.

breakfast	low-sugar granola with semi skim and berries, green tea
mid-morning snack	pot of natural yogurt coffee with milk
lunch	chicken salad sandwich, home-made tomato soup glass of water
afternoon snack	2 oatcakes with sugar-free peanut butter tea with milk
dinner	salmon, pasta, peas, spinach and pesto glass of water

This menu contains just 36g of sugar a day. Although this is still above the WHO recommended level, it gives you an idea of how some simple changes can really cut your sugar intake. It also illustrates how difficult it is to get down to 25g per day.

	Calories kcal	Carbs g	Fat g	Protein g	Sodium mg	Sugar g
Breakfast						
Lizi's – low-sugar granola, ½ cup inc semi skim	294	25	14	6	4	7
blueberries, ½ cup	41	11	0	1	1	7
Clipper, green tea with lemon, 1 mug (200ml)	3	1	0	0	0	0
Total	338	37	14	7	5	14
Lunch						
Tesco – chicken salad sandwich, 1 pack	434	45	14	31	710	5
home-made tomato soup, 2 cups	123	0	0	0	0	0
Total	557	45	14	31	710	5

	Calories kcal	Carbs g	Fat g	Protein g	Sodium mg	Sugar g
Dinner						
peas, 80g	70	12	1	5	370	4
penne, 1 cup	200	42	1	7	10	2
salmon, 1 fillet, steamed	160	0	4	23	240	0
Priano – pesto, 2 tbsp	150	2	14	2	360	0
spinach, raw, 1 cup	7	1	0	1	24	0
Total	587	57	20	38	1,004	6
Snacks						
Cooperative – natural yogurt, 125g	70	8	2	7	100	8
2 oatcakes with sugar-free peanut butter	225	14	15	8	22	1
coffee with milk	22	1	2	0	18	1
tea with milk, 1 large mug (250ml)	20	1	1	1	0	1
Total	337	24	20	16	140	11
Daily Total	1,819	163	68	92	1,859	36

How to cut back

Breakfast: 14g sugar

- When choosing your breakfast cereal, always read the label. Choose one with less than 5g of sugar per 100g. Don't be tempted by low-fat options as they tend to compensate for the missing fat with too much sweetness, and remember that even cereals claiming to have 'no added sugar' on the box can still contain too much.
- Switching from a tropical banana to locally grown berries cuts 12g (3 teaspoonfuls) of sugar from your breakfast.
- Ditch the fruit juice. Rather than being a healthy way to get more fruit into our diet, juice gives us a quick sugar hit and can contain as much sugar as a glass of fizzy pop.

Lunch: 5g sugar
- Make a big pot of home-made tomato and basil soup instead of buying fresh soup in a carton and that's another 3 teaspoonfuls less of sugar than the original lunch.

Dinner: 6g sugar
- Simply changing from sweet chilli sauce to pesto saves another 6g of sugar.

Snacks: 11g sugar
- Choosing natural yogurt cuts 16g (4 teaspoonfuls) of sugar. Although natural yogurt can take a little getting used to, it does become more palatable if you stick with it. A good way to adapt your taste buds is to start off by mixing half a portion of your usual flavoured yogurt with the same quantity of natural yogurt, gradually building up until you are able to enjoy natural yogurt on its own.
- 2 oatcakes with sugar-free peanut butter replaces the snack bar and cuts 13g of sugar.

Here are some other simple food swaps to help cut the sugar load.

	you eat this?	try this	... to cut this much sugar per portion	
breakfast	'healthy' muesli	porridge	6.6g	1.7tsp
fruit (80g)	mango	berries	7g	1.8tsp
drink	glass of juice	glass of water	21g	5.3tsp
on spag bol	ready-made pasta sauce	passata	3.7g	0.9tsp
carton fresh soup	tomato	chicken	9g	2.3tsp
biscuits	3 Jaffa Cakes	3 digestives	11.7g	3tsp

If we make these kinds of small changes, we are unlikely to notice any big difference in taste – but what we will notice is the impact that the reduction in sugar has on our health and wellbeing (not to mention the weight loss that is likely to follow).

Step 2: Eat more fat and protein

Our insulin–ghrelin–leptin cycle is in a state of chaos when we eat too much sugar (see Fat Blast, page 126, for more information). To help reverse the balance and get things back on an even keel, replacing high-sugar foods with high-fat and protein-rich foods can have a huge impact.

Just take a look at what happens to blood sugar levels when we eat carbs, protein or fat.

'To balance out sugar cravings, I eat a mixture of protein and good salads and use protein balls with coconut and cacao/nuts for a treat. It takes a while to adjust to less sugar, but you definitely feel healthier and you know you are doing better when you no longer automatically walk into the biscuit and cake aisles in the supermarket.' – EB

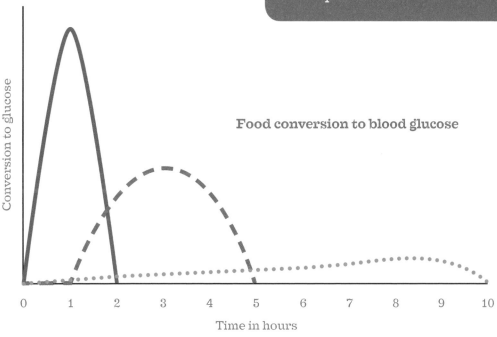

Food conversion to blood glucose

Conversion to glucose

Time in hours

━━━ carbohydrates: 90–100% turns to glucose. Peaks in bloodstream in 1–2 hours.

– – proteins: 50% turns to glucose. Peaks in bloodstream in 2–4 hours.

•••• fats: 10% turns to glucose. Peaks in bloodstream in 8–10 hours.

If you want to feel satisfied, have no sugar cravings and feel happy because your insulin has not knocked serotonin and dopamine into a state of fury, eat more fat and protein.

eat this ...	... not that
toasted coconut chips	Bounty bar
sugar-free peanut butter	chocolate spread
full-fat yogurt	low-fat flavoured yogurt
Brazil nuts	chocolate buttons

A chocolate bar may hit our reward centre faster than the coconut chips, but the coconut will satisfy a craving. Keep chocolate as a special treat rather than an everyday snack. If you really struggle to cut back on chocolate, swap to dark chocolate with at least 70 per cent cocoa solids as it can contain as little as half the amount of sugar that is in milk chocolate.

Start the day with a breakfast packed full of protein to set you up well, regulate your appetite, keep you fuller for longer and prevent the urge to snack on unhealthy foods mid-morning. For example, add a tablespoonful of nuts and seeds to your low-sugar granola, have a couple of scrambled eggs or stir some sugar-free peanut butter into your porridge.

> 'The only way I manage not to eat sugar is not to buy it.' – RM

Protein at lunchtime fuels us for the afternoon. If you usually get an energy slump around 3 p.m., take a look at what you had for lunch. Check your protein and reduce your carbs for more sustained and long-lasting energy. If you fancy a snack, then choose higher protein options to help keep you sustained. An apple and a few Brazil nuts, or some houmous on a couple of oatcakes are satisfying snacks.

Step 3: Eat fewer carbs

All forms of carbohydrate (e.g. bread, rice, pasta, breakfast cereals, crackers, biscuits, etc.) turn into glucose, but some faster than others. Low-sugar wholegrains and fibre-rich foods tend to be slow-release carbohydrates (also known as low-GI (glycaemic index) carbohydrates), while refined and sugary forms of carbohydrate are fast release or high GI. Low-GI foods provide us with a slow, steady release of energy and keep us feeling fuller for longer, without spiking our insulin levels, while high-GI foods give us an instant spike in blood sugar, resulting in increased insulin and a corresponding slump in blood sugar (and energy).

When we eat a carbohydrate-based food, our digestive system breaks it down into sugar. The increase in sugar in our bloodstream triggers a release of insulin from our pancreas to transfer the sugar for safe storage as energy in our cells, and blood sugar levels start to fall. If blood sugar levels drop, then another hormone, called glucagon, is released by the pancreas to signal the liver to start releasing stored sugar.

If we are continually eating carbohydrate-rich meals and triggering insulin, eventually our cells find it harder and harder to regulate blood sugar – our cells start to ignore the insulin message, so our pancreas produces more and more insulin and we end up with higher circulating insulin levels and higher blood sugar levels. This state is called 'insulin resistance' and is the precursor to type 2 diabetes.

If you have a real problem with balancing blood sugar, any type of carbohydrate may be a trigger for your cravings. The good carbs (low GI) and the bad carbs (high GI) can all wreak havoc with blood sugar if you are susceptible to sugar cravings. The good news is that signs of insulin resistance can be reduced or reversed by a lower-carb diet.

First, check your food diary and see which of your meals consists mainly of carbohydrates. You may find that you are starting each day with cereal and toast, having bread every lunchtime and then basing your evening meal around rice, pasta or spuds. If the thought of an entirely carb-free diet is too much to bear, then make a start by cutting back on carbohydrates at just one meal each day. Here are a few examples to get you started:

Kiwi fruit

One of the richest sources of vitamin C in our diet, kiwis are also a great source of vitamin E, folate, carotenoids, potassium and fibre. The green kiwi fruit we favour in the UK supports healthy digestion and are sometimes used as a natural laxative. Perfect as one of your two portions of fruit a day, eat them as they come or blend with other fruits and vegetables to make a delicious refreshing smoothie.

Superfoods

	replace one of these ...	... with one of these
breakfast	cereal toast	mini egg muffins with peas, feta and mint Greek yogurt with nuts and seeds
lunch	sandwich pasta salad	grilled chicken with fennel and orange salad (page 148) quinoa tabbouleh (page 151)
dinner	spag bol curry and rice	courgetti Bolognese (page 152) curry with cauliflower rice (page 153)
snacks	fruit-flavoured yogurt cheese and crackers	natural yogurt veg sticks and houmous

We have all grown up basing meals around carbohydrates in line with the healthy eating guidelines of the past, so substantially reducing carbohydrates can feel like a drastic change. But remember that we do not need carbohydrates to thrive and survive. They are not essential. The word 'essential' means our body relies on our diet providing us with those nutrients. Otherwise we simply can't survive (never mind thrive!). We need *essential* fats and *essential* amino acids (protein), but sugars and carbohydrates are not essential for life. When we eat fat and protein, we can make glucose (energy) from the macronutrients by a process called gluconeogenesis.

Step 4: Treat your treats as treats

Let's face it, a life without some little indulgence is not much fun. Rather than quitting sugar altogether, I advise that you start eating less – enjoying sugar as an occasional treat rather than a regular part of your diet.

Which takes us back to your food diary … If you find yourself edging towards the cookie jar every half hour, secretly eating a bar of chocolate on the way home and craving something sweet after dinner, then you've got it bad – but, of course, it's always possible to cut down.

If you are eating sugar:

- Five times a day, reduce to twice a day.
- Twice a day, reduce to once a day.
- Once a day, reduce to something sweet every other day.
- Every other day, reduce to twice a week.
- Twice a week, reduce to once a week.

And if you are eating sugar once a week, it is not a problem on just one condition: that any time you are munching on something sweet and sugary, you really enjoy it. Enjoy the moment, sit down, relax and savour every mouthful. As soon as you stop enjoying it, stop eating it!

Step 5: Take a supplement

Often my clients have found that taking a supplement designed to support the normal processes involved with blood sugar balance has helped them to crack the cycle of sugar cravings. The key nutrients that help manage and support blood sugar balance include:

> 'I try and make sure I don't waste my sugar allowance on something that I don't really want, that I'm just having for the sake of it, because it's in the cupboard. So, I normally buy really lovely chocolate or cake, so that when I'm having sugar it's something delicious.' – PH

- chromium – an essential trace mineral that plays an important role in regulating insulin and blood sugar levels to curb sugar cravings. Chromium is often low in our diets. Look for supplements containing chromium picolinate.
- cinnamon – it is thought that the polyphenols in cinnamon are responsible for this spice's healthy effects on sugar metabolism. As well as lowering blood glucose levels, cinnamon has been found to improve insulin sensitivity. It is often found combined with chromium in nutritional supplements designed to support the normal processes involved in blood sugar management.
- Alpha lipoic acid (ALA) – this is an important antioxidant found to be essential in regulating sugar metabolism. Its effects include reducing blood glucose levels and improving insulin sensitivity.
- Magnesium – research finds this important mineral may help reduce the risk of type 2 diabetes thanks to its effects on glucose metabolism.

> 'I also put cinnamon on my breakfast cereal to try to start the day with something which helps to balance my blood sugar.' – IM

Case study – Annie's story

When I was eating sugar I couldn't get enough. We had large tubs of Haribo in the house, and I work from home, so I regularly helped myself to some at lunchtime. I made meringues every week or two. We had cakes and biscuits regularly at social events. Bread with sweet jam, pizza with caramelised onion, hot chocolate with extra chocolate – sugar … yum, yum, yum. I wasn't overweight and my teeth were in good condition, so I didn't recognise that I had a problem.

I suffered from tiredness, though. It wasn't so debilitating that I thought it was worth getting checked out – I thought I was just lazy and that the way I was feeling was a symptom of working from home without as many stimuli around me. When I look back, though, I realise that I have always struggled with afternoon slumps, even when I was working in an office. I reached for sugar to keep me awake in the afternoons and got into a habit of grazing regularly throughout the day.

The first week I cut out sugar and refined carbs, I was gobsmacked at the lack of a slump hitting me in the afternoon. Nobody else really saw it because I would have done my best to hide it before, but I felt like I had a new lease of life. This helped to keep me on track with the diet initially.

For me the chromium supplement probably helped quite a lot at first, especially because I went cold turkey – cutting sugar out completely from the beginning. After a couple of months I started to allow myself the odd treat of chocolate, or something I really wanted, but given the changes I'd made to my diet, the chocolate didn't taste as good as I remembered. I had been missing my mother-in-law's banoffee pie and another month later I allowed myself a small slice. It was far too sweet and I didn't enjoy it. So now when I see it I'm not tempted any more.

Summary – your daily checklist for fixing that sugar fix

1. Read food labels so you know how much sugar you are eating.
2. Cut back on sugar slowly and find alternatives that you enjoy.
3. Eat more fat and protein to help you feel fuller for longer.
4. Switch to wholegrain and fibre-rich foods to help stop sugar spikes.
5. Try cutting carbohydrates out of at least one meal every day.
6. Treat your treats as treats. Eat sugar, but less of it!
7. Take a daily supplement designed to help you manage cravings.

Chapter Four

Eating For Exercise

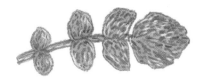

When it comes to looking after yourself, diet and exercise go hand in hand. Whether you are exercising for health and wellbeing or for competitions and performance, what you eat before, during and after training can affect recovery, fat burning and stamina. Some smart choices will help you get maximum results.

How much is enough?

Before we get down to what to eat, let's check out how much exercise is recommended each week. According to the NHS, the official minimum workout requirements for adults are 150 minutes of moderate-intensity activity like walking, bike riding or swimming (e.g. 30 minutes of exercise five times a week) OR 75 minutes of vigorous-intensity activity like jogging, aerobics or martial arts (e.g. 25 minutes of this type of activity three times a week)

Bananas

Rich in potassium, bananas are thought to improve blood pressure, water retention and reduce the risk of kidney stones. Bananas are also a dietary source of serotonin and studies have found that they may increase melatonin levels to help improve sleep quality.

Superfoods

Cacao and raw chocolate

The truth behind those headlines that tell us chocolate is good for us is that chocolate in its raw, unprocessed form is one of nature's most phenomenal ingredients. Raw chocolate (or cacao) is one of the most antioxidant-rich foods on our planet. Move over green tea and red wine, cacao contains over 300 different phytochemicals thought to exert powerful effects on our mood, heart health, nerve cell function, blood pressure and insulin balance.

Cacao is the raw, unprocessed form of cocoa powder – a far cry from the sugar-laden chocolate bars we are used to. Available as powder or nibs, cacao can be added to yogurt, baking or cereal, or used to make healthy hot chocolate (page 159). Lots of health food shops stock raw chocolate bars, but if this is a step too far then look out for dark chocolate with high cocoa solids (at least 70 per cent) as a good alternative.

PLUS strength exercises on two or more days a week that work all the major muscles, e.g. lifting weights, working with resistance bands, heavy gardening, such as digging and shovelling, or yoga.

What to eat before an early-morning training session

If you are an early bird and like to exercise first thing, make sure you are well hydrated. Drink a pint of water before your training session and sip small amounts during your warm-up and workout.

If you are planning a light session, you can probably get away without eating anything and training in a fasted state. This will help your body use fat as fuel because your energy stores of glycogen will be low, making fat the preferred energy source for your muscles.

If you are planning a heavier training session, exercising in a fasted state is likely to put your muscles under strain, making your session less efficient and harder work. For this reason, have a small snack 30 minutes before your workout to help fuel your session. This could be:

- a small pot of natural yogurt.
- apple and peanut butter.

- a plant-based protein shake with milk or almond/coconut milk. There are lots of healthy plant-based protein powders available these days, but if you prefer to make your own, check out my berry nutty shake (page 147).

Everyone is different – through trial and error you will find what works best for you.

Match your diet to your exercise

If you are trying to fit yoga classes or gym sessions into your busy week, eating the right food at the right time will help maximise the benefits of your workout. Timing your meals and balancing your carbohydrate and protein with the type of workout you do can help optimise performance, speed muscle recovery and boost fat burning.

What, when and how much to eat before and after exercise will depend on the type of exercise you do and what your goals are.

Easy training and rest days (e.g. yoga, pilates, walking)

Before exercise:

There is no need to eat anything before a session like this, but if you are peckish, have a small snack like natural yogurt and berries, or houmous with carrot sticks at least an hour before you exercise.

Eggs

Eggs are one of the most nutritious, economical and versatile foods on our shopping lists. Rich in protein, beneficial fats, selenium, zinc, iron, copper, vitamins A, E, K, B6, B12, and one of the few food sources of vitamin D, they also provide us with a unique source of fats called phospholipids. Phospholipids make up the main ingredient of our cell membranes, acting as a barrier to protect our cells from harmful intruders and helping essential stuff to pass in and out of the cells. Just make sure you eat the yolk as this is where the phospholipids are packed.

Scrambled, boiled or poached, these little powerhouses are perfect at any time of the day as a quick snack or meal. Eggs are no longer seen as the bad guys in terms of cholesterol.

Superfoods

After exercise:

Eat within one hour after your workout. A low-carbohydrate meal with some protein and omega-3-rich fats could help your muscles recover and reduce inflammation. Try something like:

- Grilled chicken and a green, leafy salad with olive oil and balsamic drizzle.
- Plant-based protein shake with your favourite milk.
- Baked salmon with roasted Mediterranean vegetables.

Low-intensity cardio exercise (e.g. jogging, swimming, cycling)
Before exercise:

If your aim is fat loss, then it may be better to exercise on an empty stomach. But remember, we are all different and some people fare better having a small snack before a training session, so try both ways to see what suits you best.

After exercise:

The debate is ongoing as to whether there is a specific window of time when we should eat after exercise. Generally speaking, aim to eat slow-release, low-GI wholegrains or root vegetables, with a protein-rich meal or snack and some omega-3 fats for muscle repair within an hour after exercise.

'I always try to exercise before dinner – the thought of dinner gets me through. I usually come home and eat a meal I prepared earlier.' – NG

If you exercise before breakfast, try my nutty granola (page 146) with Greek yogurt and berries after your session, or a couple of eggs, cooked the way you like, with toasted rye bread and grilled tomatoes.

If you exercise in the early evening, pile your plate with antioxidant-packed vegetables and some good-quality protein for dinner and eat within an hour of finishing. Try chicken with spinach and avocado salad, or make a tasty vegetable omelette with salad.

High-intensity interval training
Before exercise:

Best to train on an empty stomach, either first thing or early evening. If you've gone for the latter, leave 2–3 hours between your mid-afternoon snack and your training session and make the snack protein-based to support your muscles. A handful of nuts with an apple or pear or a plant-based protein shake would be ideal.

After exercise:
Low-GI carbs with some protein and plenty of antioxidant-rich fruit or vegetables will provide nutrients like amino acids and glycogen, and can help reduce DOMS (delayed onset muscle soreness) over the next few days. Go for something like:

- Whole baked trout (page 154) with steamed greens and a baked sweet potato.
- Mackerel on toasted rye bread with grilled tomatoes and steamed asparagus.
- Overnight oats with pear and ginger with extra walnuts (page 146).

Heavy training, endurance sport and race days

Before exercise:
Eat a carbohydrate-based meal a couple of hours before your race or training session to keep your glycogen energy stores topped up. Good choices are:

- Porridge with seeds and fruit.
- Quinoa tabbouleh (page 151) with grilled chicken.

'Before a workout I like to try and have some protein and carbs, like oatcakes and peanut butter.' – KR

Seeds

Superfoods

Seeds are little nutritional gems that have a wide variety of uses and a multitude of health benefits. From supporting healthy skin, hair and nails to lowering cholesterol, improving digestion, boosting immunity and supporting bone health, these little seeds are a must-have for health and wellbeing.

Tahini is a paste made of pulped sesame seeds. A key ingredient in houmous, tahini is packed with essential fats and protein, and contains almost three times the amount of calcium as milk. Use tahini as a spread on oatcakes, or mix with soy sauce, garlic, ginger and chilli for a marinade or dressing.

Get a variety of seeds in your diet for maximum benefits. Choose from chia, hemp, flax, pumpkin, sesame, sunflower, etc.

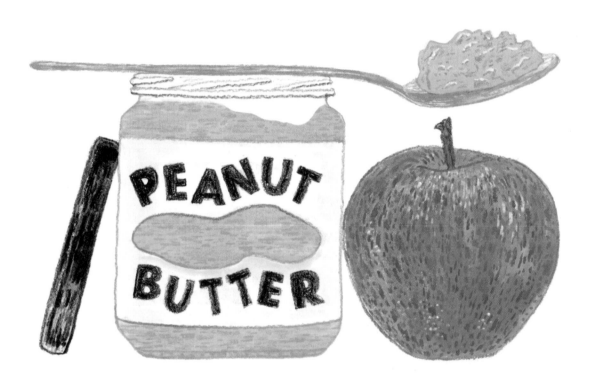

Sliced apple with peanut butter
makes a tasty and light snack
before an early morning workout.

After exercise:

Replenish glycogen stores with a carbohydrate-based meal. Try my curry in a hurry (page 153) with brown rice or quinoa.

Hydrate and rehydrate

Signs of dehydration include:

- weakness and fatigue
- headaches
- nausea
- feeling lightheaded or dizzy
- muscle spasms or cramps

If you are training when you are dehydrated, your body will tell you about it!

Whether you are exercising or not the very best way to hydrate your body is to drink water and plenty of it. Aim for a couple of litres every day and keep an eye on the colour of your pee to check if you have had enough.

Ideally, your urine should be a light straw colour. Dark yellow or brown pee usually indicates that you need to drink more water. If your pee is a bright yellow, fluorescent colour, it's probably because you are taking a multivitamin or B complex supplement – this can be a bit startling if you are taking supplements for the first time and are not expecting it!

Drink more water

If you struggle to drink enough water, these simple tips might help:

- Drink 250–500ml of water before your workout and sip from your water bottle throughout your training session.
- Every time you fill the kettle to make a cup of tea or coffee, pour yourself a glass of water to drink while you wait for the kettle to boil.
- Set a bottle on your desk and drink it throughout the day. Look for a bottle that is glass rather than plastic. Plastic has been cited as having an adverse effect on hormone balance, not to mention the environmental consequences.

- Fill a bottle with water, and then add some sprigs of herbs, like rosemary or mint, some slices of orange or lemon, or a few strawberries to give it a hint of flavour. Keep it in the fridge and enjoy it throughout the day.
- Always have a jug of water on the table at mealtimes.
- Swap one or two of your daily cups of tea or coffee for herbal tea.

Superfoods

Beetroot

This earthy root vegetable is a source of iron, folate, magnesium, antioxidants and nitrate. Recently beetroot has gained popularity thanks to its potential to reduce blood pressure and improve exercise recovery and muscle strength. Beetroot is a source of dietary nitrate which gets turned into nitric oxide in the body to help enhance blood flow and balance blood pressure.

The amount required to optimise sports performance is 400mg of natural nitrate – the amount found in a small glass of beetroot juice.

If you notice a pink or red tinge to your pee after eating beetroot, it could give you a clue that your stomach acid levels are a little low and the red pigment has not been broken down by your digestive processes. This phenomenon is known as beeturia.

My top 10 training foods

1. Salmon is packed with omega-3-rich fats to help support joints, reduce pain and inflammation in muscles, and aid recovery.

2. Anything green and leafy! Green, leafy vegetables provide folic acid and much-needed magnesium to help nourish your muscles.

3. Red meat for iron. Iron is carried around your body attached to haemoglobin. If levels are low, it's more difficult for your muscles to get enough oxygen for recovery, so you end up feeling more fatigued. Aim to have good-quality, lean red meat a couple of times a week. If you are not a meat eater, other sources of iron include dark green, leafy vegetables, dried fruit (e.g. apricots), nuts and beans.

4. Nuts and seeds are rich in vitamin E and essential omegas for joint health and muscle function. A handful a day will do the trick.

5. Oats are low GI – they provide slow-release fuel. Porridge or oatcakes are ideal on training days, but for maximum benefits add in some protein like nuts, seeds, cottage cheese or yogurt to keep you going for longer.

6. Cacao is a potent antioxidant which may help to minimise free-radical damage to tissue and reduce DOMS. One study found that a protein recovery drink with additional flavonol-rich cacao decreased muscle soreness after exercise.

7. Berries and cherries are a great source of flavonoid-rich antioxidants to aid recovery and repair after hard training sessions. Try a bowl of berries with some natural Greek yogurt and a sprinkle of cacao nibs for a post-workout treat.

8. Eggs are the ultimate protein supplement for exercise enthusiasts. They are the best source of a unique nutrient group called phospholipids, which help with mental acuity and brain function as well as sports performance and muscle recovery. Eggs are also a good source of choline, the precursor for the neurotransmitter acetylcholine, which sends messages from the brain to muscle fibres to allow muscles to contract. Choline levels are depleted with strenuous exercise.

9. Bananas have been the fruit of choice amongst runners, cyclists and sports people for years, and with good reason. They are a good source of potassium, vitamin C, B vitamins and fibre, making them an ideal post-recovery snack to rebalance electrolytes and replenish glycogen stores.

10. Sweet potatoes are a great slow-release, antioxidant-packed carbohydrate source for dinner after training.

Chapter Five

Sleep Well

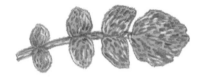

A good night's sleep will mean that you wake up feeling refreshed, revived and ready to start the day with a spring in your step. Unfortunately – in an age when technology is everywhere, being 'busy' is only ever seen as a good thing and stimulants keep us going – our sleep is suffering and insomnia is rife. Our internal body clock has lost its natural rhythm.

Our primal bodies respond to light and dark over a 24-hour period to tell us when we should be awake or asleep. This sleep–wake cycle is also called our circadian rhythm. This is why most of us feel less energetic and more tempted to hibernate during the winter months – and then spring comes and suddenly we feel more sprightly. There is a small but important pea-sized gland in our brains – called the pineal gland – that responds to daylight and darkness. When light enters our eyes, the pineal gland is switched off and the production of melatonin (the sleep hormone) is suppressed. When it starts to get dark, the pineal gland increases

'A warm bath in candlelight, lavender oil, a comfortable bed and a good read all help me to sleep well, as well as avoiding violence on TV, which often means the news too.' – SL

production of melatonin so we start to feel sleepy and ready for bed. Melatonin plays a key role in balancing and coordinating our circadian rhythm.

Levels of melatonin start to increase from early evening onwards, usually peaking between 2 a.m. and 4 a.m. and then steadily declining as morning approaches. Levels of melatonin are at their lowest levels between 3 p.m. and 5 p.m.

Most adults need about eight hours of good-quality, unbroken sleep a night. When we don't sleep well it affects our body and mind with long-term repercussions for our health and wellbeing. Disrupted sleep patterns have been linked to obesity, cardiovascular disease, depression, cravings, cancer, IBS and cognitive decline. Sleep is essential to our health and wellbeing.

Sometimes the triggers to our pineal gland can get a bit mixed up and our sleep suffers. As our pineal gland responds to light, use of electronic devices, tablets and screens can suppress melatonin and affect our sleep. Stimulants like coffee or energy drinks have also been found to reduce melatonin secretion. The feeling of jet lag is a good example of our internal circadian rhythm being out of sync with the external light–dark environment; shift workers also have to overcome the body's natural desire to be sleepy at night and alert during the day.

Superfoods

Oats

The humble oat has been found to benefit blood pressure, digestion, cholesterol, stress and anxiety. Beta glucans are found in the fibre of oats and they have been shown to help reduce both total cholesterol and the harmful LDL (low-density lipoprotein). Clinical trials show an improvement in cholesterol after just four weeks of eating oats. A couple of oatcakes, a bowl of porridge or switching to an oat-based cereal are easy ways to increase your daily intake.

What can we do to rebalance our sleep–wake cycle?

1. Switch off all electronic devices at least one hour before bedtime and never ever take your tablet or phone to bed. Blue light suppresses melatonin, so it's also a good idea to switch your devices to night-time mode or night-shift mode in the evening.
2. Electromagnetic fields (EMFs) have been shown to suppress melatonin. Our exposure to EMFs has increased with our reliance on wireless devices. To minimise

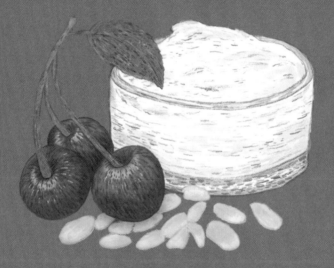

Try cherries, yogurt and flaked
almonds to help you get to sleep.

exposure it is advisable not to keep your phone or tablet in the bedroom, to switch off wireless devices and to turn appliances off at the socket before going to bed.

3. If you have a TV in the bedroom, it could be affecting the quality of your sleep. You are likely to go to sleep later and research shows that watching TV disrupts our sleep–wake cycle. For better-quality sleep and more of it, try taking the TV out of your bedroom for a month and see if it makes a difference to you.

4. Rest, relax and unwind at bedtime. Stretching, meditation, relaxation techniques or simply reading a few pages of a good book can help our minds relax and switch off – giving our brains the message that it is time to take a break and let our bodies rest.

5. Exercise helps too, as long as it's not too late in the evening. Studies show that people sleep significantly better and feel more alert during the day if they exercise regularly. It seems that exercising outside in daylight hours is particularly beneficial for toning up your pineal gland and reconnecting with your sleep–wake cycle. Save money on gym membership and get on your bike, or go for a walk in the great outdoors instead.

6. To stimulate optimal melatonin production use blackout blinds so your bedroom is in complete darkness at night. Even a small amount of light can suppress melatonin and interfere with your sleep pattern.

7. Know your stimulants. Caffeine stimulates the nervous system and increases energy, and its effects can be felt for up to five hours. So, for a good night's sleep, avoid caffeine in the evening. Try herbal teas instead – look out for ingredients like lemon balm and valerian as this combination of herbs has been shown to be particularly effective for sleep and relaxation. Tea, green

Superfoods

Yogurt

Plain natural yogurt is what I am talking about, not the sugary, flavoured stuff we have become used to. Check you are buying a live or bio yogurt to get the full benefits of the lactic acid bacteria like *Lactobacillus acidophilus* and that have probiotic effects on our gut. These essential bugs have widespread health benefits far outreaching the effects on gastrointestinal health. Some people with a dairy intolerance have found that they can tolerate live natural yogurt thanks to the probiotic bacteria it contains.

tea, coffee, energy drinks and chocolate all contain caffeine and tend to be too stimulating for a good night's sleep.

8. Eggs, fish and walnuts, tomatoes, cherries, mushrooms and cereals are some of the foods that naturally contain melatonin. The amino acid tryptophan, found in foods like oats, bananas, milk, pulses and almonds, is required for melatonin production. Increasing sources of these foods in your diet has the potential to support sleep.

9. Blood-sugar imbalance and mild hypoglycaemia can trigger your adrenals to release adrenalin to compensate for low blood sugar. Having adrenalin coursing through your body at 3 a.m. or 4 a.m. is sure to wake you up. So if you get over to sleep okay, but find yourself waking a few times during the night, try cutting back on sugar, eating fewer carbohydrates and having some protein with every meal. This will help balance your blood sugar – and you could end up with the additional benefit of a good night's sleep too.

10. A carefully chosen snack an hour or two before bedtime may help balance blood sugar and reduce insomnia. Try a couple of oatcakes with almond butter, a little natural yogurt with cherries or a couple of kiwi fruit.

11. Magnesium is sometimes known as nature's tranquilliser yet most people in the UK are deficient in it. Magnesium is found in dark green, leafy vegetables, nuts and seeds. Epsom salt baths are also a great way of topping up your magnesium levels and can help you relax and unwind at bedtime. Add a few drops of an essential oil – like lavender or camomile – to your bath then cocoon yourself in a duvet and prepare to sleep like a baby.

Superfoods

Cherries

Dark, tart Montmorency cherries are the king of the cherry family when it comes to influencing our health. With their potential to help us get a good night's sleep, recover quicker from injury and help with gout, this antioxidant-rich fruit packs a powerful punch.

It seems the most beneficial way to consume cherries is as a daily concentrated juice (with no added sugar).

'I don't think anything helps a good night's sleep more than tackling stress and anxiety.' – BM

What are you sleeping on and in?

Investing in bedding made from natural materials like cotton and wool could be money well spent. Wool pillows and duvets with cotton sheets and covers may help regulate body temperature better than down or polyester. Wool is also naturally resistant to dust mites, so it is a good hypoallergenic choice too. Look out for UK or Irish products.

> 'A warm bath, reading, lavender pillow spray and a quiet, dark bedroom.' – EAC

Sleep supplements

There are plenty of nutritional supplements that claim to be the answer to insomnia, but few that deliver results. Over the years I have tried different supplements and herbal remedies with my clients and the ones I have found to be most effective include:

- cherry extract – a natural source of melatonin found to improve sleep duration and quality.
- magnesium – may improve sleep quality and help muscles and the nervous system to relax.

Often these supplements contain additional calming ingredients like hops or L-Theanine too. Of course, rather than being the definitive answer, nutritional supplements are part of a holistic package of diet, exercising at the right time of the day, rest, relaxation and stress management to help improve sleep quality and quantity.

> 'I always sleep better when I am organised for the following day – lunches made, uniforms ready, and bags packed and by the door.' – JC

Nutritious nightcaps

A small snack 60–90 minutes before bedtime could help you catch some Zs. Try these ideas:

- Natural yogurt with cherries and flaked almonds.
- 2 oatcakes with almond butter.

- A small bowl of porridge with walnuts, cinnamon and grated apple.
- Warm milk (or warm almond milk) with cinnamon, nutmeg and ginger.

Summary – your daily checklist for sleeping well

1. Switch off electronic devices at least one hour before bedtime.
2. Do something relaxing in the evening.
3. Exercise outside in daylight hours.
4. Use blackout blinds.
5. Cut caffeine out of your diet from late afternoon onwards.
6. Eat some melatonin or tryptophan-rich foods like oats, cherries or kiwis.
7. Cut back on sugar and junk foods.
8. Sleep in and on natural fabrics.

And finally ...

If you can't sleep, get up, have a cup of herbal tea and then try going back to bed. Don't lie there counting sheep.

'If I'm feeling restless, a soak in an Epsom salt bath before bed helps.' – GC

Chapter Six

Eat Well, Age Well

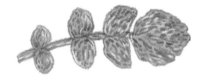

No matter what age we are, we are getting older every day as our cells are continually dividing and replicating. Each time cells divide, tiny units of DNA called telomeres get shorter. Telomeres act like the plastic tips at the end of shoelaces to prevent genetic strands from getting tangled up or fraying.

Telomere length has been used as one indicator of how well we are ageing. The good news is that nutrition can influence the rate of telomere shrinkage and therefore can help us to age well.

If we can influence telomere length, we have the potential to prevent age-associated diseases. Certain lifestyle factors like intermittent fasting, eating a diet rich in fruit and vegetables, healthy fats (from oily fish, avocados and nuts) and fibre, staying lean and active with regular exercise, and managing stress through meditation have all been shown to help reduce telomere shortening.

'Beautiful young people are accidents of nature, but beautiful old people are works of art.' – Eleanor Roosevelt

We know that lifestyle factors that promote inflammation or oxidative damage to cells – such as smoking, lack of exercise, environmental pollution, stress and unhealthy diets – increase the rate of telomere shortening. Obesity, insulin resistance,

> 'I definitely notice that I look younger when I'm eating well. Too much sugar, tea and alcohol affects my skin.' – SL

cardiovascular disease and neurodegenerative conditions like Parkinson's disease have been linked to shorter than average telomeres.

It seems that the traditional Mediterranean diet – packed with antioxidant-rich phytonutrients, as well as oily fish, olive oil, herbs and spices and sufficient sunshine to get good levels of vitamin D – plays a part in giving us long, healthy telomeres.

Specific nutrients have been linked to healthy telomeres too. Folic acid; B vitamins; vitamins D, E and C; zinc; and polyphenols like resveratrol, grapeseed extract and curcumin from turmeric are all thought to have an influence. Studies show that people who take a daily multivitamin and mineral tend to have longer telomeres than their peers who don't.

What is the elixir of life?

Rather than looking for one silver bullet for healthy ageing, we should be looking at the bigger picture of how we choose to lead our lives. If we look at populations in the world where people live long and healthy lives, there are five regions that stand out because of the number of people living there who reach their hundredth birthday and beyond. These areas are known as the 'Blue Zones' and are:

- Sardinia, Italy
- Okinawa, Japan
- Ikaria, Greece
- Loma Linda, California
- Nicoya, Costa Rica

Although these diverse populations have different diets, lifestyles and genetics, they have common characteristics that we can all learn from. They have active lifestyles and a strong sense of purpose, live in communities with good social connections and eat masses of plant-

> 'Over the years, I've noticed that happy people seem to look more youthful than those who are stressed, angry or negative. For me, a big part of "staying young" is learning new things and being open to new experience.' – NO

based foods, most of which they grow themselves. It seems that wine could also be an ingredient for longevity, as most of these communities drink wine in moderation with meals.

A lifetime of ageing well

Whatever your chronological age, you can make choices that will add life to your years. Babies and children have very specific nutritional requirements that are covered in detail in many great books, so I am going to start with nutrition for teenagers.

Teenage Dreams

Being an adolescent can be difficult, but a few changes to food and drink can make life a little easier, and help teenagers to feel and look happier and healthier. If you are the parent or guardian of teenagers, I don't advocate making a big deal out of diet, but rather think it's important to educate and inform teenagers about nutrition as much as we can. I definitely don't want to encourage dieting for this age group.

- Beauty comes from the inside out. Teenage hormonal changes sometimes cause skin to change from baby soft to stubbly, spotty or blotchy. One way to combat this is by drinking enough water and balancing the oiliness in skin with good fats from oily fish (salmon, mackerel, trout, herring, sardines), unsalted and unroasted nuts and seeds, avocado, olive oil and coconut oil. Eating less junk food, fizzy drinks and sugary sweet stuff can help too.
- Teenage girls have a tendency to be low in iron when their periods

Ginger

Ginger is packed with hundreds of bioactive compounds like gingerols and shogaols. Research indicates that ginger accumulates in our gut making it particularly effective in aiding the treatment of nausea, and as a possible colon cancer-preventing compound. It has also been reputed to alleviate the pain and swelling associated with arthritis, and has the potential to reduce the risk of cardiovascular disease and diabetes.

Superfoods

start, so eating more iron-rich foods can help combat this. Telltale signs of low iron include tiredness and lack of energy, pale skin, heart palpitations and breathlessness. Sores on the side of the mouth, a sore tongue and headaches are the less well-known signs. The best possible source of iron in the diet is red meat, but other sources include dark green, leafy vegetables like curly kale and watercress, pulses and beans, nuts and seeds, eggs, and dried fruit like apricots or prunes.

- Puberty is a time when it feels like your body is not your own. Hormonal changes can make teens feel and look different than before. Some of the most important nutrients that help support hormone balance are zinc (found in nuts, seeds, shellfish and meat), protein and good fats (from avocados, oily fish, houmous, nuts and seeds).

- Because teenagers are growing quickly they need loads of good nutrition. Most teenagers in the UK are low in vitamin A, iron, calcium, zinc and iodine.

Superfoods

Olive oil

Olive oil is a key ingredient in the Mediterranean diet – contributing to its reputation as the healthiest in the world. Olive oil is a monounsaturated fat (MUFA) and the main fatty acid it contains is called oleic acid, which has anti-inflammatory effects.

There is a big range in quality of olive oil and I would suggest always opting for organic extra-virgin olive oil if you can. It is often a darker green colour than the refined version and it is in this colour and nutty taste where we find a lot of the beneficial phytonutrients in olive oil. One of the main antioxidants, called oleocanthal, gives olive oil the gently burning taste on the back of your throat and has been attributed with anti-inflammatory properties and possible anticancer effects.

How to use:
- Choose organic extra-virgin olive oil.
- For dressings and drizzling.
- Okay to cook with as long as you don't heat it to high temperatures. It is not meant to smoke!

What is it?	Where do we get it?	Why do we need it?
Vitamin A	cheese eggs oily fish milk and yogurt liver and liver products	for cell growth and renewal healthy skin and hair eyesight immunity
Iron	liver meat beans nuts dried fruit, e.g. apricots wholegrains, e.g. brown rice fortified breakfast cereals most dark green leafy vegetables	Iron is important in making red blood cells, which carry oxygen around the body.
Calcium	milk, cheese and other dairy products dark green, leafy vegetables (not spinach) tofu nuts bread made with fortified flour fish when you eat the bones (e.g. sardines and pilchards)	helping build strong bones and teeth regulating muscle contractions, including heartbeat making sure blood clots normally
Zinc	meat shellfish dairy products bread cereal products, e.g. wheatgerm	making new cells and enzymes processing carbohydrate, fat and protein in food wound healing

- Teenagers need to move their bodies! Cycle, swim, walk, roller skate or disco dance. Exercise will help improve mood, balance weight and is the perfect way to de-stress. The NHS recommends that teenagers and young people are active for at least sixty minutes every day.
- Drink water instead of fizzy drinks. Dehydration causes tiredness, affects skin and can cause constipation. Not pretty! Teenagers – and everyone – should drink about six glasses of water every day.
- The average teenager consumes three times the official recommended amount of sugar every day. This worrying statistic is why many of our teens are overweight, not to mention the impact all this sugar has on hormones, concentration and mood. Switching from fizzy drinks to water or having healthier snacks like bananas or natural yogurt are small but effective changes.
- Keep an eye on red meat consumption. The National Diet and Health Survey has found that boys aged between 11 and 18 tend to eat too much red and processed meat. Cut back a little on processed foods like sausages, burgers and kebabs and switch to chicken, fish or turkey for a healthier choice.

In your twenties

Being a twenty-something can bring lots of change to your life. You might find yourself living away from home for the first time, getting your first 'real job' and trying to juggle all this with budgeting and partying. It can be hard to find a healthy balance.

If you can establish some healthy habits in your twenties, they will stick with you for life.

- Learn some basic recipes to set the foundations for a nourishing and healthy diet. Get into the habit of batch cooking a couple of times a week. Get a group of friends together and take it in turns to cook for each other once a week.
- Take lunch to work with you to save money and keep you better nourished, rather than relying on canteen food or eating sandwiches every day. Make soups, super salads, baked frittatas or filled wholemeal pittas for healthy, tasty and economical lunches.
- If you like to work hard and party harder, then give your liver a helping hand with foods like broccoli, cabbage, cauliflower, onions, leeks, scallions

and beetroot, and drink a couple of cups of green tea a day.

- A bottle of milk thistle complex can help to mitigate the toxic effects of the night before, but don't use it as a free pass to drink more alcohol! Alternate each alcoholic drink with a big glass of water to keep well hydrated and minimise your hangover too.

- Bone density reaches its peak in our late twenties, so make sure you are packing in bone nutrients like:

> » calcium from dairy products, nuts, seeds, and dark green, leafy vegetables.

> » vitamin D3 – may be best to take as a supplement.

> » boron, which is found in foods including nuts, avocados, broccoli, potatoes, pears, prunes, honey, oranges, onions, chickpeas, carrots, beans, bananas and red apples.

> » vitamin K2, which is found in dark green, leafy vegetables like broccoli, as well as cauliflower, vegetable oils and wholegrains like oats, barley and brown rice.

> » magnesium, which is found in dark green, leafy vegetables, nuts, brown rice, fish, meat and dairy products.

> » vitamin A – found in cheese, eggs, oily fish and liver.

> » phosphorus – found in red meat, dairy foods, fish, poultry, brown rice and oats.

> » zinc – found in meat, shellfish, nuts and seeds.

> » copper – found in nuts and shellfish.

> » manganese – found in tea, nuts, cereals and green, leafy vegetables.

Also be aware that alcohol, smoking, high-protein diets, a high intake of caffeine and certain medications – like diuretics, steroids and antacids – may impair bone health at this critical time.

Sweet potatoes

Unlike the humble spud, sweet potatoes count towards your 7-a-day target as they are classified as a vegetable rather than a carbohydrate. They have a low glycaemic index and are packed with vitamin A, vitamin C, potassium, fibre and a group of antioxidants called anthocyanins.

Superfoods

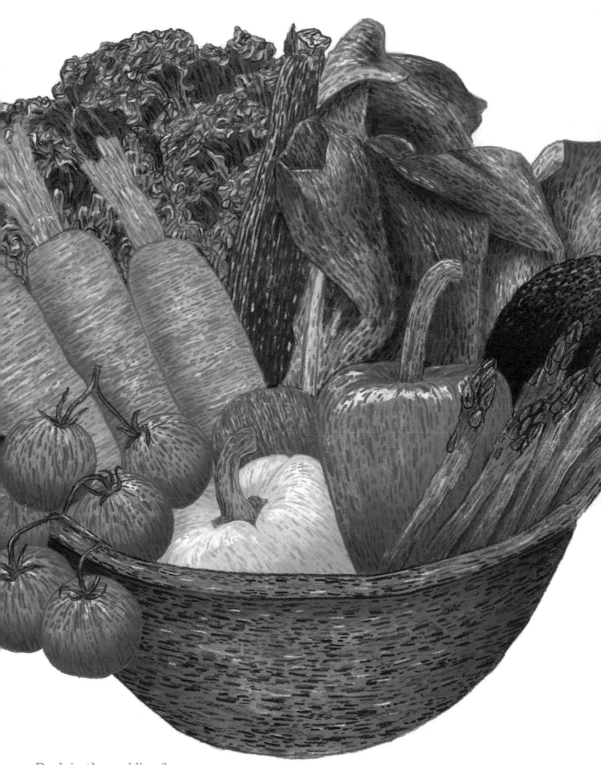

Pack in the veggies for an
antioxidant hit, whatever your age.

- Eat fish at least once a week. It is economical, packed with nutrition and fast to cook. Try white fish baked with sliced lemon and herbs, or add prawns to your stir-fry for a quick and healthy dinner. Check out my recipes on pages 154 and 155 for ideas.

In your thirties

For lots of people, being in their thirties is not much different to their twenties; while for others, it can mean settling down, buying a house, raising a family or putting more focus on career.

- If you are thinking of starting a family, top up your vitamin and mineral levels with a good quality multivitamin containing at least 400mcg of folic acid, additional vitamin D and a fish oil containing EPA and DHA.
- Eating low-sugar, high-protein snacks will help combat cravings and keep your metabolism ticking over.
- Pack in plenty of good fats for hormone balance and joint health. Avocado, oily fish, coconut oil, nuts and seeds are ideal.
- Eat some dairy produce for optimal calcium intake. Full-fat natural yogurt, cottage cheese or feta make healthy choices that tend to be well tolerated by most people.
- Keep quick snack foods in the fridge so that when you get really busy you still have healthy choices. Houmous and raw veg sticks or a hard-boiled egg with some spinach are great protein-based snacks.

Green tea

Put the kettle on, it's time for tea. The polyphenol epigallocatechin gallate (EGCG) is one of the most abundant ingredients in green tea and it is this that gives green tea its myriad beneficial effects, including fat burning, anticancer, cardiovascular health, anti-inflammatory and anti-ageing effects. As with everything in nature, it is likely that it is a combination of the plant chemicals found in green tea that make it so good for us – there isn't just one magic bullet.

Green tea also contains L-Theanine. This interesting amino acid has been found to help the brain produce alpha brainwaves which help us feel relaxed without drowsiness.

Superfoods

- Don't rely on coffee to rev up your energy levels. Instead, keep well hydrated, cut back on sugar and eat a balance of low-GI carbs and protein with every meal.

In your forties

This is when most of us start to notice some effects of ageing. Our skin is not quite so supple, we spot lines and wrinkles a little more often, our fitness levels may not be what they used to be, and our unhealthy habits start to catch up with us.

- Adjust your calorie intake a little. With each passing decade from our 40s onwards, we need fewer calories. As we age, our basal metabolic rate slows and we may notice the onset of middle-age spread for the first time. Cutting back a little on carbohydrates and stopping snacks between meals should help keep this in check, but if you want to up your game, you may find that intermittent fasting helps keep your metabolism ticking over and your weight under control. Start off eating lighter one to two days a week and see chapter ten (Fat Blast) for more ideas.
- To help keep your skin nourished and supple, take a vitamin C supplement to help support collagen production. Collagen is the most abundant protein in the body and, apart from its role in keeping wrinkles at bay, it is important for digestive and joint health too.
- Up your protein levels. If you struggle to have protein with every meal, then good-quality, plant-based protein powders made from nuts and seeds are a good choice. These are widely available and can be made into a healthy shake with your favourite milk, added to yogurt or used in baking. Grass-fed collagen supplements may help support skin health. These are usually sold in capsule form or as a tasteless powder that can be stirred into drinks like tea or coffee.
- Start taking a supplement for your joints. Turmeric and fish oil may help support joint flexibility and balance inflammation.
- Build some strength and stretching exercises into your normal routine.

'Be aware of your language and thoughts so that you stay in an optimistic frame of mind.' – LS

Nuts

Raw nuts can be a healthy addition to your diet as they contain plenty of good fats, as well as calcium, magnesium, selenium and vitamin E. One study of over 120,000 middle-aged to elderly people in the Netherlands found that those eating just 5–10g of nuts a day showed increased lifespan compared with those who didn't eat any nuts.

Sugar-free nut butters like almond, peanut and cashew are a tasty way to get nuts into your diet. Try some spread on a chopped apple or a couple of oatcakes as a healthy snack.

Nuts may also be a useful addition to your diet if you are trying to lose weight as a small handful contains fibre, protein and good fats to support metabolism, leave you feeling fuller for longer and balance blood sugar and insulin levels. Good choices include:

- almonds: protein, calcium and vitamin E
- Brazil nuts: fibre and selenium: just two Brazil nuts a day provides 100 per cent RDI for selenium for an adult
- cashews: iron, low-GI rating
- hazelnuts: fibre, potassium, folate, vitamin E
- macadamias: highest in monounsaturated fats, B1 and manganese
- pecans: fibre and antioxidants
- pistachios: protein, potassium, plant sterols and the antioxidant resveratrol
- walnuts: alpha-linoleic acid, plant omega 3 and antioxidants

Superfoods

In your fifties

Hormones may start to become an issue in our fifties when women reach menopausal age (somewhere between 45 and 55 for most women), and men's testosterone levels can start to decline. Digestion may also become an issue – stomach acid levels start to decrease, which in turn has an impact on the absorption of nutrients like vitamin B12.

- Eat mindfully. Sit at a table to eat all your meals and don't rush your food. This not only helps your digestion, but can also help to bring a sense of calm to an otherwise busy day.

- As we age, stomach-acid levels start to decline, making it harder to break down protein. Digestive issues like heartburn, wind and bloating could be down to low stomach-acid levels, so try a digestive enzyme with HCl and pepsin, available from any good health food shop.
- Phytoestrogen-rich foods like pulses, flaxseed, broccoli and chickpeas can help support natural hormone balance for both men and women.
- Foods for prostate health include oily fish, tomatoes, pumpkin seeds and walnuts.
- Look after your heart with regular exercise, and a Mediterranean-style diet featuring plenty of colourful vegetables, olive oil, oily fish – and a little red wine from time to time.
- If you don't already, start taking a fish oil supplement to support heart health, joint health and skin health. However, if you take blood-thinning medication like aspirin or warfarin, do not take fish oil supplements without consulting your GP.
- Stretch every day to help mobilise joints and prevent stiff and sore muscles.

In your sixties

As we enter our 60s, vitamin D can become an issue because older skin loses its ability to convert sunshine into vitamin D. Keep a check on your sugar intake, too, as it can increase the risk of weight gain and type 2 diabetes.

- Take a vitamin D supplement every day, especially in the autumn and winter months.
- Keep up with your regular exercise, but get outside to max up your vitamin D levels. Cycling or walking are ideal, and a great way to help you cope with the demands of a busy lifestyle.
- Make time for meals and enjoy what you eat. There is good research to show that if we enjoy the food we eat, we absorb more nutrition from it.
- Replace tea and coffee with green tea or herbal teas like peppermint and fennel to aid digestion and reduce caffeine highs.

In your seventies and beyond

Keeping fit and active as a septuagenarian will help keep your health in good nick for years to come.

- Eat your main meal at lunchtime if you can. You may find it is easier to digest.
- If you have noticed your appetite starting to decline, then eat little and often and make sure that everything you eat is packed full of nutrition for maximum health benefits.
- Soluble fibre from oats, milled flaxseed, root vegetables and fruit will help to keep your bowel healthy.
- Don't forget to keep well hydrated with water to help energy, digestion and kidney function.
- Get outside every day and keep active. Whether it is walking, cycling, yoga, swimming or gardening, physical activity will help keep you supple and has been shown to have a positive impact on mental acuity as we age.
- Keep in touch with friends and family. Social interaction is just as important to our health and wellbeing as diet and exercise.

No matter what your age or stage of life, making healthy lifestyle choices and enjoying good quality, nourishing food is the ultimate form of health insurance.

Chapter Seven

Stress Less

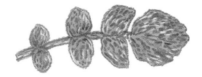

Stress and adrenalin

Stress is a normal part of life – a trigger for us to adjust or respond to a situation. It has a positive effect, making us feel alert and switched on. It's what gets us out of bed in the morning and motivates us to do things. Stress only becomes a problem when it is more than we can cope with – when we are faced with continuous challenges without any opportunity for time out to rest and relax.

As humans, we are designed to adapt to stress and learn from it. Our primal brain tells us when we are in danger or under attack and puts us into fight-or-flight mode, forcing us to decide whether to flee at top speed or stay put and fight to defend ourselves. These days we will never need to run away from a sabre-toothed tiger but the stress response is still the same – no matter whether you are fighting traffic or fighting tigers!

A short, sharp shock of adrenalin should be enough to get us moving and out of danger's way, but in the modern world we tend to run on adrenalin and have it coursing through our bloodstream for much longer than it should. This leaves us anxious, sleepless and eventually burnt out and depressed.

When we are late for a meeting and stuck in traffic, our thoughts can send a message to our brain that the situation needs action. The imminent danger of being late triggers a cascade of events in our body. Our hypothalamus gets the message to tell our pituitary to trigger the adrenals to move us out of harm's way and we are fired into fight-or-flight mode, so we end up feeling stressed and anxious about something that is not really a big deal. This complex interplay between our hypothalamus, pituitary and adrenal glands is called the HPA axis.

Our adrenal glands can only be fired up for so long before something has to give. The fight-or-flight response is supposed to be a short-lived experience. Rather than rushing from one stressor to another we need a break to give ourselves time to recover and reset the balance. If we live in a high-adrenalin state for too long (weeks, months or decades rather than seconds or minutes), we end up feeling exhausted.

Our adrenal glands sit on top of our kidneys in the small of our back, and they should be switched ON–OFF–ON–OFF/STRESS–RELAX–STRESS–RELAX rather than being on high alert all the time. Our body should have time to recover from one stressful episode before we fire something more at it.

Tomato puree, passata and tinned tomatoes

These are all a great source of of a potent antioxidant called lycopene that gives tomatoes, pink grapefruit and watermelon their pinky red colour. Lycopene is beneficial for cardiovascular health and has been linked to a reduced risk of prostate and breast cancer. It seems that cooked tomatoes are superior to raw when it comes to our ability to absorb lycopene. Add some olive oil to maximise absorption even further.

Superfoods

The stages of stress

Stress can be mental, emotional, physical or environmental. Our lifestyle habits can all add up and contribute to the stress response. When we are under pressure a cup of coffee and a chocolate bar may seem like the solution to help us feel better, but this snack could in fact add to our woes as caffeine and sugar can both send us into an adrenalin spin. Our body has the same response to sugar, caffeine and junk food as it does to stress.

Over time our adrenal glands become exhausted and we feel wiped out – but a bit anxious and wired at the same time. This is simply because our adrenal glands are out of sync with reality: they are firing off adrenalin in response to things that our bodies are perceiving as threats; even small things that might not have worried us before can make us feel stressed, anxious and out of control.

If we continue in this state for a while, eventually burnout strikes. This feels like total and utter exhaustion. Body, mind and spirit are deflated and it is a struggle to do anything.

Most of us have experienced all three stages of stress:

Stage 1
Wired. Running on adrenalin and taking on the world.

Stage 2
Wired but tired. Just about keeping going, but starting to feel cranky and exhausted. Relying on caffeine and sugar to keep going.

Stage 3
Burnout. Can't take any more. Need a holiday!

Superfoods

Avocado
Packed with healthy monounsaturated fats, antioxidants and fat-soluble nutrients, avocado has become an essential in any health-conscious shopper's basket in recent years.

Sometimes we get stuck at stage 3. This can happen after years of living on adrenalin and pushing ourselves beyond what our bodies can bear. Eventually our adrenals give up the struggle and force us to crash. Often people who have crashed go to their doctor, only for all their test results to come back clear, which leaves them searching for answers.

The good news is that with the help of nutrition and a few changes to our lifestyle, we can rebuild our resilience and resistance to stress, no matter what stage of adrenal stress we find ourselves at.

So, what's the link with nutrition?

The first thing to consider is that the food and drink we rely on to give us an energy kick could be part of the problem. A diet packed with too much sugar, caffeine and junk foods, combined with a hectic pace of life, will catch up with us sooner or later, so we crash and burn. Think about what happens to our bodies in the split second that we recognise something as being stressful.

1. We identify a stress, triggering our HPA axis to come into play and tell our adrenal glands to trigger an adrenalin rush. This increases the level of glucose (sugar) in our bloodstream.
2. Our pancreas registers the high blood sugar level and releases insulin to bring it back to a normal level.
3. The sugar is stored as fat (thanks to insulin's great fat-storage effects). Throw a little stress into the mix and cortisol directs this fat storage around our middle.
4. Before long blood sugar levels drop and the whole cycle starts again: we feel anxious or jittery and in need of a caffeine/sugar/carb fix to reset the balance (usually unsuccessfully).

Notice that the trigger for this cycle can be stress, stimulants, sugar or refined carbs and that, although the trigger may differ, the crazy sugar–stress spiral is exactly the same.

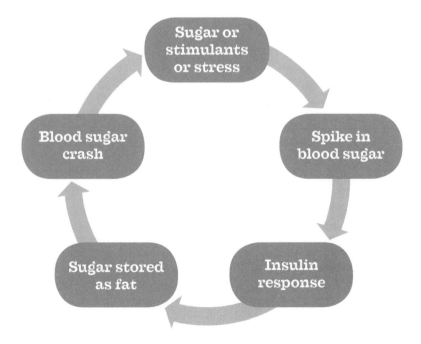

Cut sugar out of your diet for a week, and then reintroduce it and notice what happens. The chances are that you will become a bit jittery or anxious, feel your heart pounding and start craving more sugar. Exactly the same effect that stress has on your body.

The adrenal rebalance plan

'Limiting alcohol and caffeine is important for me.' – SL

So, here's the lowdown on how to rebalance your adrenals and manage stress through diet:

Step 1 – cut out sugar and caffeine

Cutting out sugar and caffeine helps to reduce unnecessary adrenalin being released in response to blood sugar fluctuations. If you are on the sugar rollercoaster and finding it hard to step off, following the sugar fix daily checklist (page 54) is a good place to start.

You could also try taking a supplement to help manage blood sugar fluctuations. Look for those that contain a combination of chromium, B vitamins and magnesium to help support sugar and insulin balance.

Step 2 – eat enough protein

When you're thinking about what to eat, start with the protein and build your meal around it. Lean meat, chicken, fish, pulses, nuts, seeds, yogurt and tofu are all good choices as they provide good-quality protein that provides your body with the amino acid building blocks to support hormone balance.

Eating a high-protein breakfast within one hour of waking can help balance blood sugar more effectively and manage early morning cortisol levels. Here are a few ideas:

- Breakfast salad: eggs, avocado, rocket, tomatoes, peppers and smoked salmon (page 145), sprinkled with some toasted seeds.
- Porridge with stewed apple and a handful of nuts (e.g. almonds or walnuts).
- Scrambled eggs with tomatoes and watercress on a slice of sourdough (rye or wholemeal) bread.

Step 3 – eat calming foods

Certain foods can have a calming effect on the body:

- Oats, almonds, avocados, pulses, chicken, turkey and yogurt contain the serotonin precursor tryptophan. We need serotonin to help us feel calm, happy and relaxed.
- Chicken, turkey, fish, milk, yogurt, cottage cheese, cheese, peanuts, almonds, pumpkin seeds, sesame seeds, avocados and bananas contain the dopamine precursor tyrosine. Dopamine gives us our drive, motivation and get-up-and-go.
- Eat your greens! Dark green, leafy vegetables are packed with magnesium, which is depleted in times of high stress. Green, leafy veg are an essential part of your recovery plan. Watercress, curly kale, pak choi, broccoli, leeks, spinach, rocket … if it's green, it's in.
- Eat oily fish at least twice a week. The omega-3 fats found in salmon, sardines, herring and trout help support and nourish your nervous system.

Step 4 – move your body

Exercise every day, but choose the right sort of exercise.

If we are at stage 1 of stress, high-intensity exercise can help release endorphins and relieve stress and tension. HIIT training, running and circuit classes are all fine, as long as you remember to breathe! Often when we are at stage one, we feel 'caught-in-the-headlights', and the adrenalin rush means our breathing can be shallow. Focus on how you breathe when exercising, and if you find yourself holding your breath or breathing through your mouth (both of which can elevate cortisol levels even further) then try to breathe more deeply and through your nose instead.

High-intensity training is definitely not the name of the game when you are at stages 2 or 3 as it will trigger more and more cortisol production and leave you totally and utterly burnt out. Walking, swimming or bike riding are all good, as long as you don't push it too hard. Take it easy and see your exercise regime as a way of relaxing and unwinding, rather than letting your competitive spirit get in the way.

Step 5 – get outside – every day!

Research proves that the great outdoors is nature's best medicine and being outside has a natural, calming effect on our nervous system. If the sun is shining, you will benefit from the extra vitamin D too. The advice for those

'There is nothing better to lift one's spirits than being in the open air.' – LT living in the UK and Ireland is to get outside for a few minutes of the day, every day, without sunscreen, taking care not to allow the skin to redden or burn – preferably wearing a T-shirt and shorts instead of covering up. Of course our climate means that this is impossible for seven months of the year, so a vitamin D supplement can top your levels up. Come rain, hail or shine, spending time in green spaces has a positive effect on mental, physical and emotional wellbeing, so get outside every day, breathe in the fresh air and surround yourself with nature as much as you can.

Step 6 – rest and relax

Meditation and prayer send our brains into a higher dimension, one where cortisol and adrenalin are out of the equation and relaxation is the priority. When we are chilled out, our parasympathetic nervous system is in the driving seat. Sometimes called the 'rest and digest' system, the parasympathetic system conserves energy because it slows our heart rate and allows us to relax.

When we give ourselves time to rest and relax, we reset our equilibrium and rebalance our adrenals. This is why mindfulness has been shown time and again to be so very effective at helping manage anxiety, depression and stress.

Step 7 – positive vibes

Dance around the kitchen, have a luxurious bubble bath, plant something in the garden … Do something that makes you feel good to help you recover from your busy day.

Managing stress

Nutrition can be a powerful tool to help you manage and cope with stress.

Stage 1: wired
anxiety, agitation, irritability, irrational anger

If you are feeling like this, then it's time to bring some calm to the situation to stop you moving into stage 2.

Follow the adrenal rebalance plan as set out on pages 88–90 plus:

1. Exercise – walk, run, cycle, spin, jog, dance around the kitchen. Just get your body moving. Remember that stage 1 is fight-or-flight, so your body is trying its damnedest to get you to move. Exercise can help to dissipate some of this

nervous energy. It doesn't have to mean going to the gym or doing an hour-long class. Think 20-30 minutes every day to move your body and burn off the adrenalin. Just remember to breathe!

2. When you have exercised you should find it easier to sleep and relax, so if you can, use the time after you have been exercising to take 5–10 minutes out. Meditation or mindfulness is ideal, but if your mind is still too active to switch off, then stretching is great too, or simply take 3 or 4 deep breaths in and out. When we are in fight-or-flight mode, our breathing tends to be shallow, so there is less oxygen available to our muscles and we can end up feeling flat and fatigued. Breathe slowly and deeply to get more oxygen circulating and your energy levels flowing.

3. Supplements that can help balance high cortisol and support you when you are feeling wired, stressed and anxious are:
    *   Lemon balm and L-Theanine. Often found together in nutritional supplements, this pair have a lovely calming effect on body and mind. L-Theanine is an extract from green tea and lemon balm is a herb from the mint family. The combination of the two has been shown to to relieve stress and anxiety, help us focus with a clear and calm mind, and support sound sleep without causing drowsiness during the day.
    *   Milk protein hydrolysate, sometimes known as lactium, has been shown to reduce stress-related symptoms and promote relaxation to improve sleep

Green, leafy vegetables

Dark green, leafy veg like rocket, watercress, spinach, Swiss chard, kale and broccoli really are the epitome of a superfood. Although not as exotic as some others, these local, homegrown lovelies really pack a punch when it comes to nutrition. Dark, dark vibrant greens are a source of magnesium, selenium, folic acid, carotenoids, manganese, vitamin C, vitamin K and fibre.

The antioxidants lutein and zeaxanthin found in green, leafy vegetables like kale, spinach and spring greens help protect our eyes against the damaging effects of UV light and are thought to reduce the risk of macular degeneration. Eat your greens!

Superfoods

quality, naturally maintain healthy blood pressure and promote healthy cortisol levels.

- Magnesium. Stress depletes our body of magnesium, and low magnesium manifests as anxiety and stress, so this one is a no-brainer. Magnesium has a calming effect on the nervous system and helps to relax muscles. Choose magnesium citrate or magnesium glycinate, as they are easily absorbed. Epsom salt baths also help us to replenish magnesium levels.

Stage 2: wired and tired

insomnia, anxiety, depression

At this crucial stage it is time to make some changes – otherwise you might burn out. Of course there are many other reasons for anxiety and depression and it is not solely down to adrenal stress, but if you feel that stress is getting the better of you, these ideas might help:

Follow the adrenal rebalance plan as set out on pages 88–90 plus:

1. Talk about it, and don't be afraid to ask for help, whether it's talking to family and friends or making an appointment to see your doctor.
2. Rest, but in an active way. Getting outside, being creative with art, crafts or cookery and walking are ideal recovery techniques at stage 2. Often people say they can't settle to meditate, so art, drawing, crosswords and anything creative will achieve the same end goal of getting you to switch off.
3. Remember what makes you laugh and try to do something that makes you happy every day.
4. Supplements that may be helpful at this time include:
   - Magnesium – to calm and relax body and mind.
   - 5HTP – to support serotonin production and improve mood (NOT to be taken with any mood-modifying medication).
   - Vitamin B complex to help nourish and tone the nervous system.
   - Lemon balm and L-Theanine to aid sleep, help you relax and improve clarity of focus.

Nourish your adrenals to balance your stress.

Case study – Lisa-Jane's story

Jane,

When I first met you in late 2015 I was feeling very low – anxious, edgy, racing heartbeat, achy limbs, headaches, and my energy levels were up and down. I had a lot of hidden sugar in my diet, I ate too many low-fat products and not enough nutritious food. In fact, I was pretty much starving myself of all the foods that I should have been eating.

So I cut down on – practically eliminated – sugar and low-fat products from my diet and I began to eat a lot more natural, unprocessed, good-quality food, and more fruit and vegetables. I cut out white carbs and now only eat wholewheat and wholegrain (apart from the odd roast potato or a few chips as a treat!). You also gave me a couple of supplements to help rebalance my adrenals. I took some magnesium and L-Theanine with lemon balm for stress and anxiety.

I always try and eat a varied diet so avoid eating the same thing two days in a row. I learned the importance of adding protein and good fats, like nuts, avocado and oily fish, to my diet to help with stress and mood. Within a couple of weeks I started to notice a difference.

I now feel a lot better – younger overall! Much more sustained energy, better mood, my edginess has gone, my heartbeat is more normal, I feel less anxious and I have fewer aches and pains. I have never eaten more or enjoyed my food more and yet my weight is spot on and never fluctuates. I am definitely a huge advocate of a healthy, nutritious diet! In addition, I also find that practising mindfulness is good for managing my anxiety. I've gone to a lot of mindfulness classes and also practise at home using apps such as Insight Timer and buddhify.

Stage 3: tired

chronic fatigue, adrenal burnout, depression

At this stage it can feel like a struggle to motivate ourselves, but there are things we can do to help us feel a little better. Be gentle with yourself and give your body and mind time and space to recover.

Follow the adrenal rebalance plan as set out on pages 88–90 plus:

1. Give your body time and space to rest and relax.

2. Epsom salt baths at least three times a week.

3. Add sea salt to your food and water sparingly – so you can taste it, no more.

4. Do a little exercise every day. Gentle stretching, yoga, Pilates, walking. Nothing too demanding, but move your body to relieve tension and generate energy.

5. Meditate every day. Try a mindfulness app, or sit outside and listen to the birds singing, smell the flowers in your garden, or just notice the different colours and textures of the plants around you.

6. Supplements that can help give you a little additional support include:
   - Siberian ginseng and Rhodiola are known as 'adaptogenic' herbs, and can work to help support and rebalance your adrenals and improve energy. Do not use these if you are taking any prescribed medication for anxiety or depression.
   - B vitamins to help tone and support your nervous system.
   - Omega-3 fish oils to help nourish and support your nervous system and balance inflammation.
   - Magnesium – to help calm and relax.

Healthy shortcuts for busy weeks

If you tend to grab food on the hop and don't think too much about eating healthy food when life gets busy, then these simple ideas will help to keep you nourished and healthy.

- Make one-pot wonders like a tasty tagine (page 156), or use a slow cooker for soups, stews and casseroles, and freeze the leftovers. Home-made soup is very restorative and a great way of packing in plenty of adrenal-nourishing foods like green, leafy vegetables.
- Pack your freezer with essentials like vegetables for roasting and frozen fillets of fish (plain ones, not breaded or battered!) for a quick and handy midweek dinner.
- Prepare some hard-boiled eggs to have with salads for lunch.
- Keep some healthy ready-made foods in your store cupboard. Pre-cooked grains and lentils can form a great base for salads or dinners, tinned fish is handy for lunch and canned beans or lentils can be added to curry, chilli or stew to give extra nutrition.

- Fish is healthy fast food when you are feeling tired or have had a busy day. Serve with salads, roasted vegetables or sweet potato wedges and frozen peas for a healthy take on fish and chips.
- Don't forget about eggs at teatime. Making a great big vegetable omelette is a tasty and quick dinner, and it can be eaten cold with salad for lunch the next day if there is any left over.
- Pick up a pot of houmous, carrot sticks, cherry tomatoes, sugar snap peas and a pack of oatcakes for a quick and healthy meal if you have forgotten to bring lunch to work.

'I've changed by being a little more organised with meals – I was at a point where I would be going for four days in a row without tea in the evenings becase I was so busy. I now prepare meals in the morning or the night before.' – JG

Summary – your daily checklist for stressing less

1. Cut back on sugar and caffeine.
2. Increase your protein levels, especially in the morning when cortisol levels are naturally higher.
3. Eat some calming foods like chicken, almonds, avocado, pulses and green, leafy vegetables.
4. Get some exercise and move your body.
5. Get outside – every day!
6. Do something that helps you to rest, relax and unwind.
7. Remember to have fun. Do something that makes you happy.
8. Take a deep breath.

One-day plan for adrenal balance

Wake up, get up and stretch your body.

Breakfast
Eat a protein-based breakfast – perhaps something like a couple of scrambled eggs with tomatoes, watercress and one slice of rye bread with a cup of green tea.

Lunch
Leftover salmon from last night's dinner, with a quinoa tabbouleh (page 151), making enough to do tomorrow's lunch with tonight's leftover chicken.

Get out for a walk after lunch to clear your head and help your mind unwind.

Afternoon
Low-sugar fruit, like an apple or a pear, with some almonds.

Dinner
Rosemary, lemon and thyme chicken (page 154) with steamed broccoli, green beans and sesame seeds, drizzled with a little olive oil and a pinch of sea salt.

Do something that helps you relax in the evening. An Epsom salt bath, reading a book or meditation are ideal.

Switch off tablets, mobile phones, TVs and screens at least one hour before bedtime.

Supper
An hour or two before bed have some lemon balm herbal tea and natural yogurt, almonds and berries.

Chapter Eight
Immune Boosters and Balancers

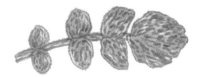

Your immune army

Immunity starts from the outside in – the first line of immune defence is formed by our skin and digestion. They act as barriers to stop pathogens invading our body and causing us harm. When something does threaten an attack, our next defence is the innate immune system, triggering white blood cells to attack viruses, bacteria and any foreign invaders. Our adaptive immune system – which is more targeted – is the third line of defence. Tailored to tackle individual threats, this specific immune response is how we build up immunity to viruses and bacteria.

Our well-armed immune system's arsenal includes cell reactions, production of antibodies, identification of rogue cells and invaders, antiviral weapons, and the ability to switch on and off our attack mechanisms to prevent our bodies reacting against themselves.

Various factors that affect our immune system include:

- calorie intake – low-calorie diets compromise our ability to fight infection.
- sugar consumption – sugar and vitamin C compete for absorption by our cells and compromise our immunity. Even natural sugars like honey have been shown to deplete immune function and prolong illness, so those cough

sweets and honey and lemon drinks might best be avoided at the onset of a cough or cold.

- stress levels – negative emotions and high stress levels are linked to a lowered immune function.
- gut microbiome – the ecosystem of our gut helps defend us against pathogenic microorganisms and plays an important role in balancing our innate and adaptive immune responses.
- exercise – while excessive exercise can have a negative impact on our immune system, moderate regular exercise like walking an hour a day could help give us an immune boost.
- alcohol – affects immune function and depletes us of nutrients like zinc and the B vitamins that are required for immune support.
- sleep – helps us repair and recover from illness: white blood cells are generated while we sleep.
- vitamin D levels – all immune cells have vitamin D receptors, making it a key nutrient for immune function. People living in the UK and Ireland are at risk of low vitamin D levels between November and February due to our shorter days, cloudy weather and lack of sunlight. Research shows that vitamin D levels are at their lowest in February, which coincides with the highest incidence of colds and flu. It is advisable to use a vitamin D supplement and to have your levels checked regularly. You can access vitamin D testing through City Assays http://www.cityassays.org.uk/vitamins.html.

> 'I'm a great believer in resting when you are ill. Nourishing soup with lots of healthy vegetables works for me too' – EB

- air pollution has been linked to increased inflammation and a depleted immune system.

Prevention is better than cure

The good news is that we can eat our way to a stronger immune system. Eating plenty of colourful fruit and vegetables, aromatic herbs and spices, some oily fish, and nuts and seeds is one of the best ways to support and nourish our bodies and protect ourselves from illness. There are some foods in particular that have super powers when it comes to our immune systems.

Anti-inflammatory

- colourful fruit and vegetables
- green tea
- turmeric
- ginger
- oily fish
- nuts and seeds
- tomatoes
- olive oil
- green, leafy vegetables
- fruit, especially apples, berries and cherries

Antibacterial

- garlic
- lemon juice
- oregano
- manuka honey
- apple cider vinegar
- fermented foods like live yogurt, sauerkraut, kimchi, etc.
- coconut oil
- oregano

Antiviral

- garlic
- berries (especially elderberries)
- ginger
- chicken soup
- fermented foods like live yogurt, sauerkraut, kimchi, etc.
- green tea

- Vitamin A is essential for the proper functioning of our thymus gland, and of the mucus membranes that line our mouth, nose, sinuses and GI tract. The best sources of vitamin A are liver, butter, eggs and oily fish. Beta carotene is a vitamin A precursor found in green-, red- and orange-coloured fruit and vegetables.
- Selenium is also essential for immunity and to help fight infections. Selenium comes from oily fish, asparagus, beef, turkey and chicken.
- The thymus gland acts as the commanding officer of our immune systems – and zinc is an essential mineral for the function of the thymus gland. Good sources are beef, lamb, seeds, oysters and shellfish.
- Garlic – with its antibacterial, antiseptic and antifungal effects, garlic is a vital ingredient for immune balance. Eaten raw or in a capsule, research shows that garlic is a good preventative medicine against coughs, colds and chest infections during the winter or as a natural fast-acting antibiotic if we do get an infection.
- Berries are a tasty way to help support your immune system to defend your body against viruses, especially if you choose blueberries, cranberries and blackcurrants. It is thought that the antiviral effect is due to the high polyphenol antioxidant levels that these berries provide.
- When it comes to boosting our immune systems, citrus fruits are often the first thing we think of. They have a reputation for being high in vitamin C – although, in fact, red peppers contain more vitamin C than oranges. However, it is possible that it's more than just the vitamin C in citrus fruit that gives our immune systems a boost. Powerful bioflavonoids, including a

> 'I eat more onions and garlic – I definitely think this helps fend off illness.' – LA

Berries

Blueberries, strawberries, raspberries, blackcurrants and blackberries are the richest sources of some of our most potent antioxidants including proanthocyadins, flavonols, ellagic acid and resveratrol. Attributed with improving cardiovascular health, reducing neurodegenerative oxidative stress and their ability to act as anti-inflammatories, these tasty little gems are one of the jewels in our fruit bowl.

Superfoods

Superfoods

Bone broth

Homemade bone broth or stock – made by simmering bones for several hours, often with apple cider vinegar, some bay leaves and a few vegetables (like carrots, onions, leeks and celery) – is packed with nutrition and has a soothing effect on the gut thanks to its high gelatin or collagen content. For my recipe, see page 158.

Superfoods

Citrus fruit

Grapefruits, oranges, lemons and limes may do more for your health than just adding a pop of flavour. These zesty citrus fruits are packed with antioxidants with exotic-sounding names like hesperidin, nobiletin, naringin and tangeretin, that are thought to support liver health, have anticancer properties and work like natural antibiotics.

Buy unwaxed citrus fruit and use the zest in cooking as this is where a lot of these bitter-tasting phytochemicals are found.

substance called Hesperidin which is found in the pith of citrus fruits, have strong antioxidant effects and help to maximise the effects of vitamin C. Hesperidin has also been shown to have an antihistamine effect.

- Mushrooms are renowned for their immune-boosting capabilities, but it is often the maitake, reishi or shiitakes used in Asian cuisine that claim the glory. Our common white, button and chestnut varieties tend to be overlooked but they contain compounds with powerful immune-balancing and anti-inflammatory effects too.

- Fermented foods like live yogurt, sauerkraut, kimchi and kefir help keep our friendly gut bacteria in balance. These lactic acid bacteria have been shown to have therapeutic effects on the immune system, including benefits for allergies, eczema and viral infections.

- Quercetin – found in apples, onions, berries, brassica vegetables, capers, shallots, tea and tomatoes – may help us fight infection thanks to its wide range of biological actions including anti-inflammatory effects, natural antihistamine properties and the potential to reduce pain from inflammation.

- Eat a rainbow! The more colourful the range of fruit and vegetables you can eat, the better for your immune balance.

For example:

» Berries and cherries
» Dark green, leafy vegetables
» Orange-coloured fruit and vegetables

Get well soon

Taking regular exercise, eating a nutritious diet and keeping stress levels in check are some of the best ways to help support the lines of defence we have against a cold or virus, but if you do end up with a cough, cold, snots and sniffles, there are things you can do to help yourself to get well soon.

1. Get some rest! While you sleep, you generate white blood cells which will help you get well.
2. Organic fruit and vegetables (and their skins!) provide a source of beta glucans – a type of polysacchardies found on the cell walls of fungi and yeast that have been shown to reduce the effects of a cold or flu and get you back on your feet sooner.
3. Keep well hydrated with enough water.
4. Eat plenty of herbs and spices, especially garlic, ginger and turmeric.
5. Chewable zinc lozenges have been shown to reduce the severity and shorten the average cold or bout of flu by about seven days.
6. Elderberry is available as a nutritional supplement and has been found to shorten the duration of colds and flu thanks to its antioxidant, antiviral and antimicrobial properties. One study demonstrated that people taking elderberry at the onset of flu started to recover 4 days earlier than those who did not.

Superfoods

Turmeric

An essential ingredient on any spice rack worth its salt has got to be turmeric. Best if you can get it in its root form rather than as the powdered form, this bright yellow spice has anti-inflammatory, antioxidant, anti-carcinogenic, anti-ageing, mood enhancing, circulatory and analgesic effects thanks to its active ingredient curcumin.

Unfortunately curcumin is notoriously hard for us to absorb, so this may be one where supplement action with the extract is in fact more beneficial. For optimum benefits, find one that contains black pepper extract too as this pair act synergistically.

7. Don't forget vitamin C, which is often depleted when we are run-down. Vitamin C may reduce the duration and severity of your cold. It is almost impossible to get the levels of vitamin C that will help us fend off a cold from our diet, so supplementation is advised.

8. Echinacea is another immune-boosting favourite that has been well-researched. It has been shown to have antimicrobial and antiviral effects, helping to prevent the common cold and reduce its duration.

9. Eat chicken soup. Proper, old-fashioned, home-made broth has been shown to be one of our best defences against the common cold. Researchers have been slurping their way through bowls of soup to discover whether this tasty remedy is more than just a feel-good food. It seems to have positive effects on the microscopic hair-like cilia that line our respiratory tract, ears and lungs and help us to flush out mucus. When bones are cooked down to make soup, they leave behind a

Superfoods

Apple cider vinegar 'with mother'

Apple cider vinegar is one of those ingredients my grandmother had as a staple in her larder – as much for its health benefits as for its use in cooking.

Research shows that apple cider vinegar offers powerful benefits for our health and wellbeing. When choosing apple cider vinegar check the label says 'contains mother' or 'with mother' as this means you are buying the live version of this fermented food. You can see this as a cloudy sediment at the bottom of the bottle. Just give it a shake before use. Some of the benefits of apple cider vinegar include antifungal, antibacterial effects and antioxidant effects; improved blood glucose response; increased satiety; cholesterol balance; and blood pressure reduction.

How to use it:
- Mix with olive oil, mustard and seasoning to make salad dressing.
- Combine with soy sauce, ginger, garlic, chilli and a little honey as a marinade for meat, fish or chicken.
- Add a dessertspoonful to warm water and drink before meals as a digestive tonic.

Eat a rainbow! Pack as many different coloured fruits and vegetables into your diet as you can to help support and balance your immune system.

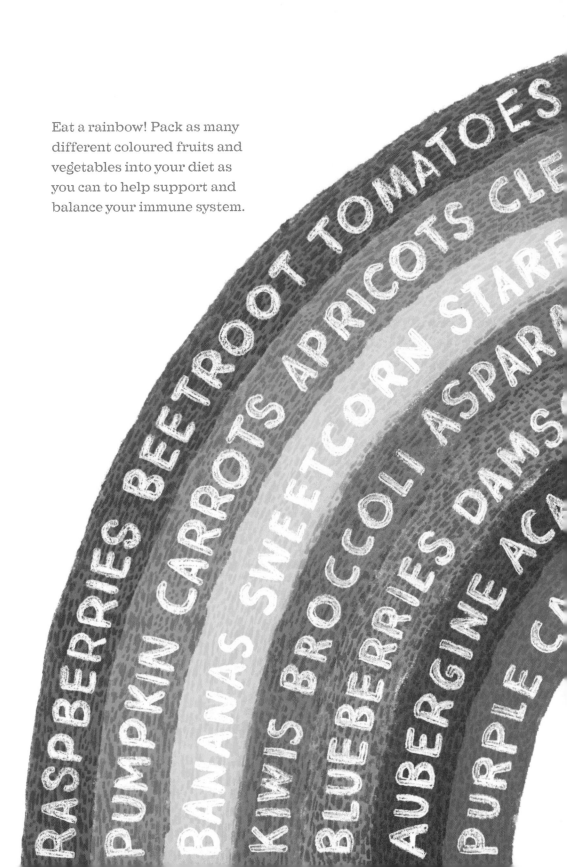

nutrient-rich broth packed with easily digestible protein, vitamins and minerals that have been found to reduce congestion, boost our immune systems, support healthy digestion and act as an anti-inflammatory. Adding some garlic, onion, leeks and vegetables to your soup will help maximise the benefits. See page 158 for my proper chicken stock recipe.

> 'If I have a cold, I'll make chicken soup. And drink lots of water – that's it really.' – DM

Balancing inflammation

The inflammatory response is an important defence mechanism employed by our immune system when tissues are injured. Our cells trigger the release of chemicals like histamine, and prostaglandins to isolate whatever has caused us harm, and trigger white blood cells called phagocytes to kill the invader.

In some conditions, such as arthritis, asthma and eczema, the inflammatory response becomes chronic and has problems switching off, causing the body to fight against its own cells. Chronic, low-grade inflammation is thought to be at the root of most of today's long-term debilitating health conditions – from Alzheimer's disease and obesity to heart disease, cancer and depression.

When it comes to supporting and nourishing our immune systems, whether to help us recover from infections and colds or to balance an overactive immune response with autoimmune conditions, addressing inflammation is a priority.

Triggers for increased inflammation:

- red meat
- sugar
- refined carbohydrate
- corn and vegetable oils
- trans fats e.g. margarine

Superfoods

Kelp and dulse

You may not find these in your store cupboard, but they were a traditional part of our diet for generations.

Packed with trace minerals they extract from the sea, these sea vegetables are a good source of calcium, iron and iodine and are making a comeback not least because they have been found to support thyroid function.

Anti-inflammatory foods

- omega-3-rich oily fish
- herbs and spices – especially cloves, ginger, turmeric and rosemary
- orange-coloured fruit and vegetables (e.g. sweet potato, butternut squash, cantaloupe melon, carrots)
- dark purple or red berries and cherries
- dark green, leafy vegetables
- avocados
- extra-virgin olive oil (for dressings and drizzles, and cooking at lower temperatures)
- coconut oil (ideal for cooking with)
- nuts and seeds (walnuts, chia, flax, almonds, etc.)
- garlic

'The first thing I do is cut out all sugars – even though all I want is a bit of comfort food, it's definitely the worst thing for me.' – RM

Superfoods

Tomatoes

When in season, tomatoes are a delicious addition to our diet and a lovely source of the antioxidant lycopene (see tomato puree, passata and tinned tomatoes, page 85, for more details). Always drizzle your tomatoes with a good-quality olive oil to max up your lycopene absorption (and to make them even more delicious). Choose organic as tomatoes are on the 'Dirty Dozen' list (page 33).

One of my favourite ways to serve tomatoes:

- Roughly chop lots of organic tomatoes (any size, shape and colour) and put them into a bowl.
- Tear up a great big handful of basil and add that to the bowl too.
- Drizzle a healthy glug of olive oil and add some freshly ground black pepper and a touch of sea salt.
- Leave to marinade for at least 20 minutes.

One-day plan for immune support

Breakfast
Overnight oats with pear and ginger (page 146). A cup of green tea.

Lunch
Home-made chicken and green vegetable soup.

Snacks
Super green smoothie.
A handful of nuts and seeds with an apple or nectarine.

Dinner
Baked fish parcels with steamed broccoli spears and sweet potato wedges.

Summary – your daily checklist

1. Rest, take it easy and get more sleep.
2. Keep well hydrated.
3. Slurp some home-made soup.
4. Pack in colourful fruit and vegetables.
5. Eat plenty of onions and garlic.
6. Drink herbal teas containing ginger, echinacea and/or elderberry.
7. Avoid smoking, sugar and stress as all three compromise our immunity.
8. Get your vitamin D levels checked and take a supplement during autumn and winter months.

Chapter Nine

Chew, Digest, Absorb

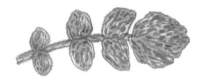

It's easy to take our digestion for granted, especially when we're younger – eating any crappy food that takes our fancy and trusting that our gut will take over, ensuring efficient digestion and absorption of nutrients. It is not until something goes wrong and we experience discomfort, pain or our toilet habits change that we start to pay our gut any attention.

We all know what it feels like to have an off day caused by digestion problems. Most of us have suffered from constipation, belly ache, heartburn, loose stools or bloating at some point – but if you are constantly suffering from these kinds of symptoms, they become debilitating and can leave you feeling exhausted, annoyed and frustrated. If you have difficulties with your digestive system, the food you eat can be a trigger for pain, discomfort and angst.

How do we digest?

Digestion starts even before we eat our first mouthful of food – the anticipation triggers our salivary glands to start releasing saliva, so our mouth starts to water at the thought of the tasty morsel we are about to enjoy. The release of small messaging molecules that are critical for digestion, such as cholecystokinin, somatostatin and neurotensin, have been found to increase by over 50 per cent just at the mere sight and smell of food. This release of saliva sets off a cascade of activity within our digestive tract. Our brain tells our stomach to get ready to digest, our pancreas is primed to release enzymes to break down our food into a form that can be absorbed by our body, and our whole digestive system gets ready to spring into action so we can efficiently digest, absorb and benefit from the nutrients in our food.

How do you eat?

If you grab a quick bite on the run, eat breakfast standing up, munch your lunch in the car or at your desk, slump on the sofa with a tray on your lap at teatime, or sit hunched over a breakfast bar, you could be laying the foundations for digestive problems.

Our digestive system is affected by our nervous system, and if our brain is not primed and ready for food, our digestion has no idea that it is about to be hit with a belly-load of food. The vagus nerve, which connects our belly to our brain, needs to be switched on to get us ready to digest. As you read in chapter one, our vagus nerve is the dominant nerve of our parasympathetic nervous system, or our rest-and-digest system, so even the name itself indicates how important it is that we sit down, get ready to eat and take our time to enjoy our food. When we are in our fight-or-flight mode, digestion is the last thing on our brain's to-do list.

Having a 'gut feeling' and 'trusting your gut instinct' are terms we use to describe the gut–brain connection. This superhighway that connects our gut to our brain is a connection of nerve cells and hormonal cues providing feedback on the state of play in our body. The messages send information back and forth about how hungry we are, how stressed we feel or if we have eaten something our body doesn't agree with. Scientists have

Superfoods

Brown rice

One of the world's most popular staple foods, this gluten-free grain is packed with soluble fibre, B vitamins, magnesium, manganese, phosphorus and selenium. The fibre and protein in brown rice make it an ideal choice for a low-GI diet. Studies have linked nutrients in brown rice with reduced risk of type 2 diabetes, cardiovascular disease and obesity. The soluble fibre in brown rice also helps to support digestion.

nicknamed this primal connection between our gut and brain as our 'second brain'.

So, never mind what you are about to eat, let's first of all think about how you are going to eat it:

- Get off the sofa and away from your desk and always sit at a table to eat – no exceptions! When sitting at a table, we are in the optimal posture for digestion. Sitting slumped over a tray or our desk, we are not.
- Switch the TV off! Watching telly as you eat triggers your fight-or-flight response system and switches off your rest-and-digest system.
- Before you wolf down your first mouthful, take a few seconds to anticipate your meal. The thought of food makes our mouth water and this production of saliva starts a whole orchestra of events designed to enable your body to successfully break down, digest and absorb whatever food you fancy.
- Take your time. It is not a race. Sparks are not meant to fly off your knife and fork. Try setting your cutlery down between each mouthful. Although this will feel a little awkward to start with, it will certainly slow you down and will soon feel like a normal habit.

Fennel

This aniseed-tasting vegetable has many uses – fennel bulb is used as a vegetable or salad ingredient, the seeds as a herb and the leaves can be infused as a tea. A good source of bone-supporting nutrients like calcium, magnesium, potassium and vitamin K, fennel has also been shown to have phytoestrogenic effects, which may enhance its bone-protective properties as well as making it a key ingredient for assisting with female hormone balance. Fennel seeds and infusions are traditionally used as a digestif and as a traditional remedy for wind and colic.

Superfoods

The process of digestion

As food passes through our digestive tract, complex mechanical and chemical reactions break it down into its basic component parts to provide us with the nutrients we need to survive, most of which we absorb in our small intestine. Once we get what we need from our food and the microbes in our gut have taken what they need and transformed the rest, it is eliminated as waste.

What is normal?

Gurglings, grumblings, farts and poo. As children, we find the topic of digestion hilariously funny, but as we get older it becomes a taboo subject and not something to discuss in polite company.

Ideally, your poo should be easy to pass and sink slowly into the toilet bowl, and should be a mid-brown colour. Although the smell will not be lovely, neither should it be repulsive.

How do you poo?

My friend Ali is a Pilates teacher and physiotherapist who is fascinated by how our posture affects our bodies and minds. Ali introduced me to the idea of having a pile of books in the bathroom – not to read, but to prop up your feet so you are in the right posture for efficient elimination.

In parts of the world where people squat, there are far fewer instances of IBS, constipation, diverticulitis or haemorrhoids. The way we sit on the loo inhibits our puborectalis muscle, meaning we don't get to eliminate efficiently and are more likely to be constipated. The answer? Put your feet up when you are on the loo.

Your good gut checklist

1. Drink up! Your digestive system needs water. Drink 6–8 glasses of water every day for optimal digestion. Herbal tea counts towards your intake, so try peppermint (a digestive aid, but may not be the best choice if you suffer from heartburn), fennel (for wind and gas) or ginger tea (for an upset tum and nausea).

2. If your digestion is sluggish and you suffer from indigestion or bloating, you may benefit from cutting back on, or even avoiding, all raw foods for a couple of weeks. So instead of salads, fresh fruit and stir-fries, try soups, casseroles and stewed fruit (without added sugar). Because the cooking process helps to break your food down, it can give your digestive system a bit of a helping hand.

	Insoluble fibre	Soluble fibre
What does it do?	adds bulk to your stools and helps things pass through more quickly	softens stools, gets things moving and keeps you regular
How will it help my digestion?	helps with constipation	helps with constipation, diarrhoea, reflux and indigestion
Where can I get it?	wholegrains skin and peel of fruit and vegetables nuts and seeds green, leafy vegetables peas and beans sweetcorn	fruit vegetables (especially root veg) brown rice flaxseed oats psyllium chia nuts

3.   Know your fibre. There are two different types of fibre in our diet – insoluble and soluble – and each has different effects on our digestion. Some people with very sensitive digestive tracts can find it difficult to tolerate insoluble fibre, which acts like a scrubbing brush on our gut and can be too much if your gut is inflamed or irritated. This is why wheatgerm, green, leafy vegetables and pulses can aggravate digestive problems in some people. Try these simple ideas to increase your fibre intake instead:

- Eat more root vegetables like sweet potato, carrots, parsnips and butternut squash (which contain more easily digested soluble fibre), and fewer green vegetables, sweetcorn and peas (which contain more insoluble fibre).
- Eat a couple of portions of fruit every day – apples, berries and kiwi are especially high in fibre. You may find that these are easier to digest if they are cooked a little. Try stewed apple, berry compote or poached pears which can be made without adding sugar. Fruits should be cooked without skin or seeds. Avocados tend to be well tolerated, but avoid bananas if constipation is a problem.
- Add a spoonful of chia or flaxseed to an oat-based cereal like porridge or low-sugar granola for a fibre-packed breakfast.

- If you suffer from constipation, try soaking 1–2 teaspoonfuls of chia, flaxseed or psyllium in a glass of water for an hour or so. Then drink the mixture, plus another big glass of water. It might not taste the best, but it should help to get your bowel moving!
- Use vegetables in creative ways to increase your intake e.g. spiralised vegetables instead of pasta, sweet potato wedges instead of chips, butternut squash instead of lasagne sheets, or grated carrot to bulk out curries and bolognese.

4. Eat or drink something bitter at the start of each meal. Traditionally, bitter foods like lemon, chicory, grapefruit, rocket, kale, watercress, radicchio or endive have been used as digestive aids. You can get similar effects from:
   - a mug of hot water with a slice of lemon or a spoonful of apple cider vinegar added to it (this is not suitable if you suffer gastritis, acid indigestion or heartburn).
   - serving watercress, rocket, radicchio, chicory or kale salad as a starter before your main meal.
   - digestive bitters in water to get your juices going. Available as a tincture from good health food shops, these mixtures often contain herbs like fennel, meadowsweet, and gentian.

5. Include some natural antimicrobial foods in your cooking, such as garlic, cloves, olive oil, turmeric, apple cider vinegar, coconut oil and oregano – a delicious way of incorporating some natural antibiotic properties into a meal.

6. Old-fashioned bone broth or stock is packed with collagen, an essential ingredient to help heal the gut. If you have a chicken carcass or some beef bones left over from Sunday lunch, strip off all the meat, and then simmer the bones with a few bay leaves, some celery, carrot and some apple cider vinegar for several hours. You can find my recipe for proper chicken stock on page 158.

7. Pineapple and papaya contain natural enzymes called bromelain and papain, which may help you break food down more effectively.

8. If wind is an issue, try eating fennel as a vegetable or salad ingredient, and chewing fennel seeds as a digestive aid after dinner.

9. Stewed apple could have particular benefits for your gut. The polyphenols and pectin in apples support the gut environment, rebalance healthy microbes and may calm inflammation.

10. Eat some prebiotic foods to help your probiotic bacteria thrive. Prebiotic foods, containing fructans and galactans, pass through your digestive tract without being broken down by stomach acid or digestive enzymes, and only become active when they reach your colon, where they provide fuel for your probiotic bacteria. A healthy balance of prebiotic foods has been shown to change the microcosm of your gut by feeding the right sort of bugs. Specifically, it seems that the probiotic genus bifidobacteria and lactobacilli thrive on a diet rich in prebiotic foods. Sometimes seen as FOS (or fructooligosaccharide) on the ingredients list of your probiotic supplement, here are some foods that have prebiotic properties:

    - apples
    - asparagus
    - banana
    - chicory
    - flaxseed
    - garlic
    - Jerusalem artichokes
    - leeks
    - onions
    - oats
    - psyllium

    BEWARE! If these foods are not a regular part of your diet, introduce them slowly. Although they are great at supporting your healthy gut flora, they can cause excess wind and bloating if you eat too many too quickly.

11. Get cultured … Fermented foods like kimchi, kefir, sauerkraut, live yogurt

Superfoods

Parsley
Curly or flat-leaf parsley is a nutritional hit. Shown to help relieve bellyache, improve heavy periods and high blood pressure, and help with water retention, parsley has far-reaching health benefits. It is really easy to grow and so versatile. It can be added to most savoury dishes or used to replace basil in pesto recipes.

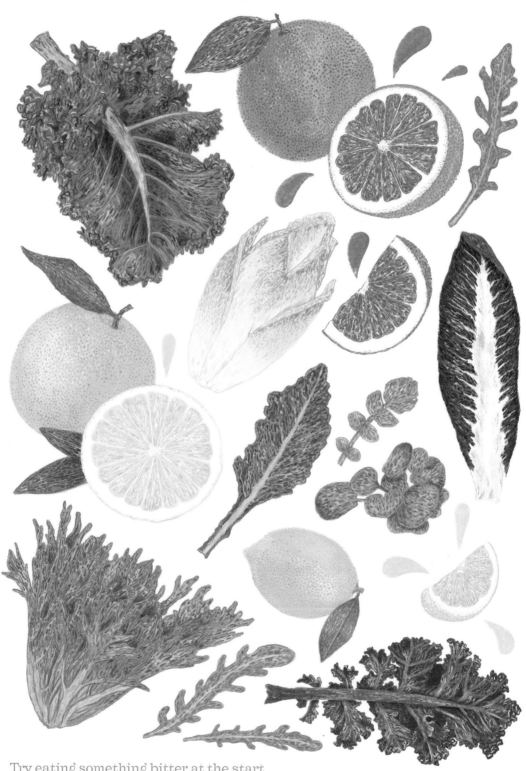

Try eating something bitter at the start
of a meal to improve your digestion.

and kombucha help keep your digestive system in tip-top health. Packed with beneficial lactic acid bacteria, these foods are natural probiotics. Introduce them gradually to your diet so you don't get windy! See my recipe for red cabbage and orange kraut on page 157.

12. Old-fashioned remedies like prunes, cabbage juice and slippery elm still stand the test of time when it comes to digestive health and regulating bowel movements.

Foods to avoid

1. Beware of high-fat foods as they may trigger constipation, diarrhoea or acid indigestion.
2. Keep alcohol to a minimum and keep at least a couple of days every week alcohol-free.
3. If you suffer from acid reflux, take a break from acidic foods like tomatoes, lemons, vinegar and apples for a few weeks to see if it helps.
4. Keep an eye on your sugar and refined-carb intake, as both will throw your good bacteria out of balance, and are often the trigger for heartburn, indigestion and constipation.
5. If you are having problems with your digestion, I suggest looking at your food diary to try to link what you are eating with how you are feeling. Remember that some digestive reactions can have a delayed onset.

Here is some more information on some of the common culprits.

Fermented foods ...

... like kefir, sauerkraut (see my recipe on page 157), kombucha and kimchi are one of the best ways to up the ante on your probiotic intake. These cultured foods are bunged full of lactic acid bacteria to help keep your gut happy.

We know that the health of our gut microbiome impacts on our gastrointestinal health but it also has repercussions far and wide in the body. From mood and memory to cholesterol and inflammation, healthy gut flora are the hidden gems of wellbeing. Watch out for pasteurised versions of these foods as they don't contain the healthy bacteria.

Superfoods

- Wheat – found in bread, couscous, pasta, biscuits, wheat bran, etc. – may seem innocuous enough, but can be a trigger for digestive problems. Look at your food diary to see how often wheat features. If you notice that you are eating wheat with most meals, then do some detective work and cut it out to see how you feel. Keep a daily food diary so you can track your progress.

replace this ...	... with this
bread	100 per cent rye bread or wheat-free bread
couscous and pasta	brown rice cauliflower rice (but not if you suffer from gas, wind or bloating) quinoa spiralised vegetables
wheat-based breakfast cereals	porridge low-sugar oat granola (page 146) overnight oats (page 146)
flour	cornflour or wheat-free flour
biscuits	oat biscuits
crackers	oatcakes

- Soya milk and yogurt have become a big part of our diets in recent years, but sometimes our digestive system finds it hard to cope with this relatively new, over-processed food. Keep an eye on food labels and try replacing soya milk with coconut or almond milk, and soya yogurt with coconut yogurt. Just check that you are buying the unsweetened version of these foods.
- Some people find dairy products – like milk, cheese, yogurt and cream – tricky to digest. Use alternatives for a couple of weeks to see how you fare.

replace this ...	... with this
milk	coconut or almond milk (check it is unsweetened)
cheese	houmous (but not if you suffer from gas, wind or bloating)
cream	coconut cream

- Other foods that have a tendency to be difficult to digest include grains, peanuts, eggs, corn, beef, pork, citrus fruit, sugar and refined carbohydrates.

'Bloating now seems to be a thing of the past. I think it was triggered by too much bread.' – JMcC

How to do an elimination diet

When cutting any food out of your diet, view the process as a short-term experiment. Even if you feel a lot better without the foods you have eliminated, they may not all be causing you a problem. For example, if you have eliminated dairy and feel much better, you may discover that you can tolerate butter and yogurt but not milk and cream. Or, if you eliminate wheat and notice an improvement in your digestion, you may work out that you can eat pasta but not bread.

If your digestive difficulties are being triggered by a particular food, a food diary and a methodical approach will enable you to track down the culprit.

Here's what I would suggest:

1. Keep a food and symptoms diary to help you discover any potential food triggers.
2. Take the suspected food out of your diet for 4 weeks. Be as strict as you can about eliminating this food entirely from your diet – check all food labels, for example, and take care if you are eating out.
3. Reintroduce the food after 4 weeks, but do this in an organised way. For example, if you have cut out dairy, then don't go crazy on cheese, milk and yogurt all at once. Instead, list all the foods you have eliminated and make yourself a reintroduction plan, leaving 4 days between reintroducing each food, and keeping a note of what you have introduced and any symptoms over the next 24–48 hours.

Day 1	Try a couple of spoonfuls of natural yogurt
Day 5	Try some goat's cheese
Day 9	Try a glass of milk
Day 13	Try some cottage cheese, etc.

Keep going until you have reintroduced all the foods you had cut out.

If you react, avoid the offending food for another 4 weeks and try the reintroduction phase again.

If you don't react, continue to reintroduce the food gradually back into your diet.

Of course, cutting any food out of your diet means you have the potential to be lacking in some nutrition, so take care to replace the food you have eliminated with something that contains similar nutrients to avoid deficiencies. For example:

Avoiding this	you need more of this	from this
dairy	calcium	sesame seeds, tahini, dark green, leafy vegetables, nuts and seeds
wheat	fibre	fruit, vegetables, nuts, seeds, oats, rye

N.B. If you are pregnant, underweight or have a history of eating disorders, do not attempt an elimination diet.

A note on the low FODMAP diet

The name FODMAP comes from the names of the carbohydrates that are restricted in the diet: fermentable oligosaccharides, disaccharides, monosaccharides and polyols. Developed in Australia, the low FODMAP diet has become very popular and, for some people, is a very effective method of managing IBS. It should not, however, be considered a long-term approach.

'I used to get really bad IBS cramps but I haven't had these for at least 10 months, just from reducing my sugar intake and cutting out refined carbohydrate, cereals, etc. Making these simple changes has dramatically helped the bloating and pain.' – PS

The low FODMAP diet uses the idea that eliminating foods with prebiotic activity will alleviate wind, gas and bloating, and indeed there are plenty of research studies to back this up as a short-term intervention.

The problem is that the low FODMAP diet restricts the intake of foods that actually support and benefit our digestion, and over a long period of time, this has the potential to knock our lovely healthy gut flora out of balance, with unknown consequences for long-term health and wellbeing.

If you are undertaking a low FODMAP diet, I would advise a supplement plan that helps support gut health, ideally including a good-quality probiotic and a digestive enzyme preparation, with a view to reintroducing the foods after time.

Low acid or high acid?

Our stomachs are basically a big bag of acid – hydrochloric acid, to be precise. This acid breaks down proteins, so we can digest them, and it kills off potentially pathogenic bacteria so they don't cause us harm.

Often when someone visits a GP with reflux, heartburn or indigestion, the first line of action is to prescribe an antacid or proton pump inhibitor like omeprazole or lansoprazole. However it is worth noting that the digestive discomfort associated with high stomach acid can feel very similar to low stomach acid, so sometimes these medications don't deliver the desired results.

Here are some common signs of discomfort associated with low stomach acid levels:

- feel full quickly after eating
- heartburn
- indigestion
- reflux
- bloating, belching or flatulence immediately after eating
- undigested food in stools
- diarrhoea and/or constipation
- acne and rosacea
- rectal itching

As we age, stomach acid levels tend to decline rather than increase, so antacids are not always the best solution.

Ghee

This clarified butter has a high smoke point, making it suitable for cooking. It is lactose free, a source of the fat-soluble vitamins A, D and E and contains butyric acid, which may support gastrointestinal health.

Superfoods

Case study – Beverley's story

After many years of fluctuating between a constant dull ache in my stomach and chronic abdominal pain, I got referred to gastro at the hospital, who couldn't find anything untoward at all (thankfully!). But this left me back at square one – all this pain and no answer as to what was causing it. Come August 2016, I spent a week in Wales in such discomfort that it overshadowed the whole holiday. Coming home from the airport I found myself almost bent over double in agony, and I decided there and then that I needed to do something. So I looked up your website to see if you held any clinics, and my journey to better health was set in motion.

What did you change in your diet?

Strangely, I found the simplest change you prescribed to be the most immediately effective – not snacking between meals. Even though I only ever snacked on things like unsalted nuts, seeds, prunes and dried apricots, I found that giving my gut enough time to digest what I had already eaten was one of the first breakthroughs.

You also advised that I cut out pork (heavy on the digestion), cut down on sugar and bake certain fruits instead of eating them raw (raw pears and apples can sometimes leave me in pain).

Did you take any supplements?

I took a digestive enzyme, L-Glutamine powder, berberine and grapeseed to help rebalance my gut flora, and a probiotic.

What triggers do you avoid?

I couldn't pin down a food source per se, although I learned it's best for me not to follow meat with fruit. My biggest triggers are two things which can be difficult to bypass – stress and a bra! Both can cause almost immediate discomfort and the removal of both can cause an equally immediate abatement. Also, I find neither overeating nor undereating beneficial. My gut doesn't like either extreme much.

What foods or drinks help you digest?

Sauerkraut, kimchi, green tea, fennel tea, etc. – bitter foods – and small amounts of quality red wine or dark chocolate help too. There's the cloud's silver lining, right?!

Take the burp challenge

There is a simple way you can discover whether your stomach acid levels might be a little on the low side. This is not an accurate science, but at least will give you an indication of where you are on the acid scale.

The theory is that by mixing an acid (the hydrochloric acid in your stomach) with an alkaline (baking soda), carbon dioxide will be produced, which makes you burp. If your stomach acid levels are on the low side, then gas is less likely to be produced and you will not burp.

This test should be used as a guide and not a definitive answer.

Stir a level teaspoonful of bicarbonate of soda into a glass of water and drink the mixture on an empty stomach. Notice how long it takes you to burp. Repeat daily for 3 consecutive days.

If you burp, the chances are that your stomach acid levels are okay.

If you are not burping after 5–10 minutes of drinking the bicarbonate mixture, you may have low stomach acid. Try taking a dessertspoonful of apple cider vinegar in water before meals, or supplementing with HCL and pepsin to see if you start to feel a little better. Never come off any medication without talking to your GP first.

The link between gut health and immune balance

Autoimmune conditions like vitiligo, rheumatoid arthritis, lupus and MS could have their origins in your gut.

The lining of our small intestine is semi-permeable so that we can absorb nutrients from our food, but sometimes these microscopic holes get bigger, allowing larger particles – like proteins, bacteria and gluten – to penetrate the gut wall and enter the bloodstream. These larger molecules set off an immune response, sending alarm bells that a foreign substance has entered our body and we need immediate immune action NOW!

Unfortunately when this happens, the holes get bigger, more particles enter the bloodstream and our immune system is primed to react. This phenomenon is known as 'leaky gut' and is thought to be a trigger for many autoimmune conditions, thyroid issues, joint problems and inflammation, as well as affecting absorption of essential nutrients like zinc, iron and B12.

Leaky gut can affect many areas of the body and the impact is often experienced as:

- constipation and/or diarrhoea
- food sensitivities
- joint pain or swelling
- skin problems
- headaches
- bloating or abdominal pain
- fatigue
- thyroid imbalance
- digestive problems
- weight gain
- blood-sugar imbalances
- allergies like asthma and hay fever
- mood swings, confusion and poor memory

It's thought that leaky gut can be triggered by some medications, antibiotic use, high stress or trauma, chronic inflammation, imbalanced gut flora or chemotherapy, but even the natural process of ageing can affect the permeability of the gut lining.

The protocol to help support the integrity of the gastrointestinal tract often focuses on the Functional Medicine model called the 5R Approach. This is:

1. **Remove** foods and factors that are contributing to the imbalance.
2. **Replace** with healing foods, digestive enzymes or stomach acid.
3. **Reinoculate** the gut with beneficial probiotic bacteria like fermented foods and probiotic supplements containing lactobacillus and bifidobacteria.
4. **Repair** the gastrointestinal barrier with specific nutrients and foods like L-Glutamine and bone broth.
5. **Retain** healthy gut function by eating well, taking regular exercise, managing stress and ensuring good-quality sleep.

The advice in this chapter will help you get a head start on the 5R Approach, but working with the support of a registered nutritional therapist or functional medicine doctor can help you to address the underlying causes of your digestive problems and develop a programme of support specific to your requirements.

One-day plan for digestive support

Breakfast
Porridge made with equal parts water and coconut milk, topped with one tablespoonful of milled flaxseed and some stewed apple with ground cinnamon. A cup of fennel tea.

Lunch
Home-made chicken broth.
Walk after lunch to help your body rest and digest.

Afternoon
A small pot of live natural yogurt or some kefir (not low fat and not flavoured).

Dinner
Whole baked trout (page 154) with roasted vegetables.
Eat dinner at least three hours before bed to give your body time to digest.

Fennel tea in the evening.

Summary – your daily checklist for digestive health

1. Get off the sofa, away from your desk and sit at a table for all your meals.
2. Slow down when you are eating and chew your food well. Setting your cutlery down between each mouthful will help.
3. Drink enough water.
4. Cut back on sugar and refined carbs.
5. Eat more fibre from vegetables, nuts, beans, lentils, flaxseed and chia.
6. Cut out wheat and dairy to see if it helps.
7. Eat some fermented foods.
8. Try herbal teas like fennel or peppermint.

Chapter Ten

Fat Blast!

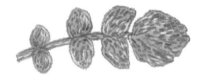

Calorie counting or intermittent fasting? Low GI or low fat? When it comes to diets for weight loss, there is so much choice that we can end up dazed and confused about the best way to lose weight and keep it off.

There is no such thing as one-size-fits-all when it comes to weight loss, but there are some simple rules that will help most of us lose a few pounds and get to our own healthy weight.

Over the decades we have seen different diets come and go as nutritional research dictates and our lifestyles change. From the F-plan diet to clean eating and beyond, there have been so many variations on the theme that it's no wonder we are a nation of yo-yo dieters looking for the easy way to get skinny.

Instead of going for a quick fix, get fit for summer or lose 10lb in 10 days plan, a more healthy attitude to weight loss is to view the food we eat as a way of enhancing our health and wellbeing. Then the issue of weight tends to become less of a problem because we are choosing food that makes us feel good, which just so happens to be the same food that helps balance our weight and metabolism. Once we get more in tune with what our body wants and needs, we usually find that some days we feel more hungry than others, and most likely these are the days when we are more active.

The calorie question

The idea of counting calories has led to such crazy ideas as cutting back on the amount of food eaten during the week to allow for a binge or booze fest at weekends; avoiding nutritious foods like avocados, nuts and seeds because they are 'fattening'; and choosing over-processed low-fat products instead of healthy, nourishing food.

The theory of calorie counting is a little outdated now, as it is thought too simplistic for the complex and individual needs of our bodies. Calories come from the three macronutrients in our diet, namely protein, fat and carbohydrate, and each of these has specific functions in our body.

Just so we can make a comparison, imagine we have:

- one single calorie from fat
- one single calorie from protein
- one single calorie from carbohydrate

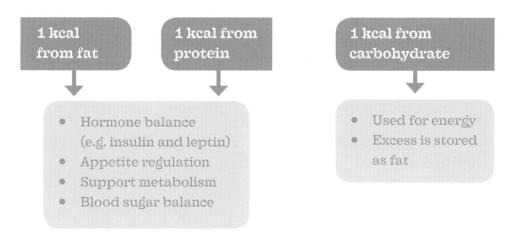

The calories we get from fat and protein help play a key role in regulating our appetite and supporting metabolism, while the calories we get from carbohydrate are the body's preferred energy source. While all three nutrients are important in our diet, healthy-eating guidelines have encouraged us to steer clear of fats and overindulge in carbs, knocking our macronutrient balance off-kilter.

It is no coincidence that since the advent of low-fat dieting, our waistlines have got wider and, as a nation, we have become fatter. Often low-fat foods are packed with sugar to make them appetising. Sugar is of course empty of any nutrition apart from being a source of fast-release energy, which eventually gets stored as fat if we don't burn it off.

Hunger hormones

Let me introduce you to ghrelin and leptin. These are sometimes referred to as the 'hunger hormones'. These two buddies work together to help regulate our appetite and influence our body weight. Although we have known about these two hormones for several years, our understanding of their function and effects is just beginning. What we do know is that this couple sends messages to our brain to signal when to eat and when our energy stores are full enough.

Ghrelin is produced in the stomach before we eat to tell our brain we are hungry and to trigger our appetite to encourage us to eat. Levels of ghrelin are suppressed for about 3 hours after eating to leave us feeling satiated.

Leptin is made by the fat cells in our bodies' stores. It helps suppress our appetite by sending a signal to our brain that energy stores are sufficiently full and we don't need any more food. In theory, the thinner we are, the less leptin circulating in our blood, and the fatter we are, the more leptin there is around. However, we can overcome and ignore the leptin message that is signalling us to stop eating. It seems that if we become overweight or obese, the leptin signal is not heard as loudly by the brain and its appetite-suppressing effects are reduced. This is called leptin resistance.

To help manage ghrelin and leptin balance, research highlights 4 key things that we can all do:

1. Eat more healthy fats
2. Eat sufficient protein
3. Eat less sugar
4. Get a good night's sleep

'Do not buy junk and choc – if it is not in the house, you will not eat it.' – JMcC

Notice how important fat is to regulate our hunger hormones. You might recognise this if you have ever tried a low-fat or calorie-restricted diet and became ravenous.

A history of dieting

Think about how food production and consumption has changed in the last 50 years. In the 60s and 70s most of us made food at home, rarely ate out, ate fewer processed foods and had smaller portions.

The yuppie decade of the 80s led to more fast food, eating on the go and our portion sizes became supersized. Bigger portions, bigger plates and bigger packets.

Have a look at how some portion sizes have changed over the last twenty years and therein lies part of the reason why our body shape is changing so rapidly.

How have portion sizes changed?

The British Heart foundation's 2013 report found that portion sizes of pre-prepared meals had generally increased over the preceding 20 years

	Margherita pizza	Family-pack salted crisps	Individual chicken pies
1993	200g	100g	160g
2013	250–460g	150g	240g

Weight loss that works

Unfortunately a 4-week diet is not going to fix a lifetime of bad choices. As you will know by now, my view on diet is that food is powerful stuff and we can eat our way to a lifetime of good health by making some simple changes to the food we eat.

Adopting some of the healthy habits I have outlined in previous chapters is likely to have the welcome side effect of weight loss, but there are a few additional ideas that can help too:

1. Time your meals

In recent years, much has been written about intermittent fasting, with diets like 5:2 or 16:8 gaining popularity. Intermittent fasting is currently hailed as the holy grail of effective weight loss. Rather than being a fad diet, it seems that the research into intermittent fasting and evidence for its success is impressive.

The gist of the science is that by subjecting our bodies to periods without food, we help balance insulin and blood sugar levels, improve leptin sensitivity and can support effective and long-term weight loss.

Of course, like every diet, there are pros and cons of intermittent fasting and different viewpoints on the best way of translating the science into real-life diets. In my experience, the simple approach is the best, so here are a few guidelines to get you started:

Step 1: know your limits

If you have any medical conditions, always check with your GP before starting any diet.

Superfoods

Butter

No buts, it's got to be butter. Throw out the margarines and low-fat spreads and get back to butter. Not only does it taste better, but this unprocessed, traditional, local, natural food has been an essential ingredient in our diet for generations and may have some hidden health benefits.

Butter is churned and made from the fat of milk, making it one of the few sources of butyric acid in our diet. Butyric acid is a short-chain fatty acid that acts as a fuel source for our gut, with potential benefits for IBS and inflammatory conditions of the gastrointestinal tract.

In the UK and Ireland most of our butter comes from grass-fed herds making it one of the very best sources of a type of fat called CLA (conjugated linoleic acid) that has been linked with fat burning and immune modulating effects.

Butter has a high smoke point, too, making it safer for cooking than most delicate plant-based oils.

It is not advisable to try this type of diet if you are pregnant, breastfeeding, diabetic or have a history of eating disorders.

Step 2: establish a low-GI diet as your healthy baseline

Before embarking on your 'fast' diet, it is important to establish a low-GI diet as a foundation for maintaining blood sugar balance and supporting your health (see Sugar Fix, chapter 3, for full details).

Step 3: eat within a 12-hour window

If you are new to intermittent fasting, the easiest way to start is by restricting your food intake to a 12-hour window e.g. between 7 a.m. and 7 p.m., or 8 a.m. and 8 p.m. Start off by doing this a couple of times a week and gradually build up to four or five days a week.

'I think low-GI works best, and eating enough, as then the cravings for chocolate and cakes reduce and eventually stop.' – GC

Give it a go to see if it suits you. Build it up slowly and if it doesn't suit you, stop!

2. Manage your carbohydrates

Rebalancing carbohydrates and thinking about when to eat carb-rich foods like potatoes, rice, pasta, noodles, bread, biscuits or crackers may help with weight management. Eating carbs earlier in the day, with breakfast and lunch, and cutting them out after 5 p.m. may help support weight loss as we will have less carbs to burn off in the evening (when many of us are less active anyway) and will be inclined to eat more vegetables. Note: you do not have to eliminate carbs all together.

instead of this ...	... try this
spaghetti	spiralised vegetables
mashed potato	butterbean and parsley mash
lasagne sheets	butternut squash or leeks
rice	cauliflower 'rice'
couscous	quinoa
bread	there is no alternative, so eat less of it!
crackers	flaxseed crackers

3. Portion distortion

Use this ready reckoner to make sure you are on track for portion sizes:

A healthy, balanced breakfast:

Take your breakfast bowl, split it in three and aim for:

- one-third protein (e.g. eggs, nuts and seeds, natural yogurt)
- one-third low-GI carbs (e.g. oats, wholegrain cereals)
- one-third fruit or vegetables (e.g. berries, tomatoes, avocado)

Pack a healthy lunch:

Eat lunch about 5 or 6 hours after breakfast (around 1 p.m. if you have breakfast at 7.30 or 8 a.m.).

Fill your lunchbox with:

- one-half vegetables or salad
- one-quarter protein (like eggs, meat, fish, chicken, pulses, feta or cottage cheese); a helping about the size of your palm
- one-quarter low-GI carbs or root vegetables (like sweet potato, beetroot or carrot); a helping about the size of your fist

A balanced dinner plate:

Avoid carbs after 7 p.m. Make creative use of more vegetables instead.

If you have supersized plates, it's time to go shopping. Using a slightly smaller dinner plate will help reduce portion size.

Fill your plate with:

- two-thirds vegetables (including at least one fist-size portion of green leafy veg). Be creative with your vegetables. There are lots of ideas in the recipes chapter, and think too about different ways of cooking them – roasting, stir-frying, poaching, spiralising all work brilliantly, and there is masses of inspiration online. Don't forget to season – a drizzle of olive oil, some sea salt and some ground pepper can transform any vegetable into something altogether tastier.
- a palm-size portion of protein.

A healthy way of eating should be with you for life – it's not just a quick fix.

4. Eat meals not snacks

Eat enough at breakfast to keep you fuelled until lunchtime and pack a lunch that will sustain you until your evening meal. This way you are less likely to crave snacks to make up for what is lacking. Remember that protein and fats help regulate our appetite and manage leptin levels, so aim to eat some of these with every meal for effective weight loss.

When I look at people's food diaries, I am often surprised by how little people eat at lunchtime. A small pot of yogurt and some fruit, a bowl of soup or a quick sandwich is unlikely to satisfy us for long, and will trigger hunger and sugar cravings mid-afternoon. Our lunch is a main meal and should be more or less the same size as dinner.

5. Cook your own food

We don't really need research to tell us that the food we cook at home tends to be better for us than the food we grab on the go – and it can help with weight loss too.

'Something I've done for decades is that, if I'm really hungry, I eat my next meal a bit early, rather than have a large sweet snack between meals. If I still want a treat after my meal, it tends to be small, which it wouldn't have been if I'd had it first.' – KL

Superfoods

Chilli

Chilli peppers are packed full of capsaicinoids, the active ingredient that has been found to exert multiple physiological effects including pain relief, control of inflammation and weight loss. Their thermogenic properties help us to expend more energy and stave off hunger, so we tend to eat less.

- Make and take your own lunch to work at least four days a week. Make it easy on yourself by using leftovers or making food in bulk that will do two or three lunches. Make up super salads, mini egg muffins or soups in bulk for weekday lunches (see recipe section for details).
- Never cook for just one meal – think leftovers for tomorrow night or next day's lunchtime.

6. Think about drinks

Fizzy drinks, cordials, alcoholic beverages and sugar in our tea all add up to potential weight gain. If you are tempted by the healthy image of fruit juices and smoothies, bear in mind that there can be as much sugar in a glass of juice as there is in a can of Coke.

Water can also help us to manage our appetites. It's easy to confuse thirst with hunger, so before you reach for something to eat, it's always a good idea to have a glass of water first, and see if that beats the craving.

7. Move your body

Diet alone will not move our muffin top, thin our bingo wings or get rid of our belly. Exercise is essential. Aim to get your body moving for thirty minutes every day.

Although the most important thing is to move, it seems that short bursts of higher-intensity training throughout your workout may help promote fat burning.

This could mean integrating some hills into your walk, running a bit faster every other kilometre, or checking out YouTube for some ideas for HIIT training.

The key is to make it work for you.

- Do something you enjoy.
- Do it with a friend.
- Schedule exercise into your busy diary.

Superfoods

Buckwheat and quinoa

These gluten-free 'pseudograins' have grown in popularity as we search for alternatives to pasta and rice in our diets.

Quinoa is one of the few vegetarian foods containing all nine essential amino acids, making it a 'complete protein'. Packed with trace minerals, and good sources of calcium, magnesium and fibre, these grains can increase variety and enhance your nutritional intake.

Here's how to cook them:

- Rinse in a sieve under cold running water.
- Put into a saucepan with 2 parts water to 1 part seed.
- Simmer for 10 minutes (quinoa) or 15–20 minutes (buckwheat).

One-day menu plan

8 a.m., Breakfast
Toasted pumpernickel rye bread with avocado, smoked salmon and cottage cheese.

1 p.m., Lunch
Super salad with last night's leftover rosemary, lemon and thyme chicken (page 154).

4 p.m., Snack (optional)
If you need a snack, have an apple and 3 or 4 Brazil nuts.

7.30 p.m., Dinner
Baked fish parcels with herby steamed vegetables (make enough to have some leftovers tomorrow).

Summary – your daily checklist

1. Time your meals. Eat all food within a 12-hour window, leaving 12 hours for your body to fast.
2. Manage your carbohydrates. Eat carbs at breakfast and lunch, but not dinner.
3. Reduce portion sizes.
4. Eat meals, not snacks.
5. Cook your own food.
6. Think about drinks.
7. Move your body every day.

Chapter Eleven

Supplement Your Diet

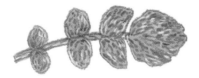

Why take a supplement?

Walk into any health food shop and you are guaranteed to be overwhelmed by the array of supplements on offer. So do we really need supplements, or are they a scam to get us spending money on more stuff we don't really need?

As a nutritional therapist my philosophy has always been food first, but I also know that the food we eat is not as rich in essential nutrition as it was 40 or 50 years ago. Thanks to intensive farming methods our soil has become depleted of nutrition and the strains of crops, chosen for their ability to grow strongly and quickly, are less nutrient dense than the species we had in our diets years ago.

One study found that over the course of fifty years, between 1940 and 1990, our food lost an average of:

- 49 per cent sodium
- 16 per cent potassium
- 24 per cent magnesium
- 46 per cent calcium
- 27 per cent iron
- 76 per cent copper

Olives

Olive oil gets the limelight, but olives are also a good source of healthy monounsaturated fats, vitamin E and antioxidants. Green olives have a higher content of polyphenols, so are best for their antioxidant content.

With all this in mind, I think there is good reason for taking a few carefully chosen supplements as part of our nutritional health insurance plan.

I would never advocate taking a supplement in place of what is lacking in our diet. Instead think of supplements doing the job it says on the tin, i.e. to supplement a healthy diet and help maximise our nutritional intake.

Price is an issue when it comes to choosing supplements and this is one area in which you really do get what you pay for. Pile-'em-high, sell-'em-cheap supplements tend to end up as expensive urine: the inorganic forms of minerals – like oxides and sulphates – used in these cheaper supplements are inexpensive to produce but are not particularly well absorbed by our bodies, so we end up peeing most of the supplement's nutrients out.

I would recommend popping along to your local independent health food shop or researching online so that you know you are buying good-quality supplements at a reasonable price. Some of my favourite brands are Viridian, Wild Nutrition and Terranova.

What to take

To keep things simple, I have pared down the lot to give you the low-down on the essentials, with a simple guide to help you decipher whether you are getting a good-quality supplement or wasting your money.

As a good baseline, I would suggest that most people could benefit from taking at least a good-quality multi-nutrient complex, and some high-strength fish oil every day. Pregnant women have specific nutritional requirements, so should choose a supplement specially formulated for use in pregnancy.

1. A hard-working multi-nutrient complex

Here's your checklist for choosing a good multi-nutrient complex:

- Is it in capsule form instead of a tablet? Tablets tend to be harder to digest.

- Is your supplement free from fillers and binders? Check the label for stuff like magnesium stearate, titanium dioxide, talc or shellac. These are fillers that your body has to process and metabolise.
- Look out for the words ascorbate or citrate after the names of minerals like zinc, iron and magnesium. These words indicate a natural form of the mineral that tends to have higher rates of absorption.
- Methylated Bs? It is estimated that somewhere between 30–60 per cent of us have problems with the methylation process, one of the most critical metabolic processes in our body that underpins health and wellbeing. Methylation is like a spark that helps to activate enzymes and prevent harmful build-up of toxic or dangerous molecules. To be sure that your multi is effective, check your B12 is called methylcobalamin. Some super-duper multis have methylated folate too (sometimes called 5-MTHF).
- Food-state supplements mirror how nutrition works in nature by combining basic nutrients with food extracts and phytonutrients to help maximise absorption and function of the formulation. This type of supplement tends to list food ingredients like alfalfa, spirulina, bilberry or turmeric.

2. A high-strength fish oil

It is impossible to ignore the vast amount of well-documented research about omega-3 and its powerful benefits for cardiovascular health, brain function, eye, skin and joint health to name a few.

Asparagus

Asparagus has a very short harvest season, so is best eaten in May and June.

Known as a hangover cure, asparagus's reputation for liver protection is due to its ability to upregulate the liver enzymes needed to detoxify alcohol. Research has also highlighted asparagus's antidepressant effects.

Some people notice asparagus's effects on their pee soon after eating – this distinctive odour from asparagus metabolites can be smelled by some people but not others. It is thought that we all excrete the same metabolites but that some people are just 'nose blind' to the smell.

Superfoods

Fish in the diet is a good idea, but a fish oil supplement helps bring additional benefits. Before you part with your hard-earned cash, do a bit of detective work to find out if you are getting a goodie.

- Is it environmentally sustainable and ethically sourced? Ideally fish oil should come from small fish like anchovies and sardines that are low down the food chain – they tend to be more sustainable and less affected by pollution.
- Is it clean? Reputable supplement companies are scrupulous about supplying sustainable fish oil from clean sources. The price you pay for higher-quality supplements means you are more likely to be buying a supplement that has been screened for PCBs, dioxins and other pollutants.
- Is it fresh and pure? Look deeper into how your fish oil is produced to ensure you are buying the good stuff. Fish oil is very delicate and can be easily oxidised, so you want the best quality you can get in a stable form. Often manufacturers add antioxidants to fish oil supplements to produce a more stable fish oil formulation.
- How much DHA (docosahexaenoic acid) and EPA (eicosapentaenoic acid) does it contain? Studies show that benefits are found in fish oil supplements containing at least 250mg of DHA and EPA.

3. Plant-based antioxidants

For extra cellular protection it is worth considering an antioxidant as part of your supplement plan. The basic antioxidants (vitamins A,C,E, zinc and selenium) are a good baseline, but a really good-quality antioxidant supplement should also pack in additional plant-based ingredients like turmeric, green tea, bilberry or grapeseed extract to harness the power of plants.

4. Vitamin D – liquid sunshine

According to UK national surveys, more than 1 in 5 of us living in the UK are suspected of having a vitamin D deficiency, with risk likely to be increased:

- the further north we live.
- the more we stay out of the sunshine.
- the darker colour our skin tone is.
- the older we are.

Think about food first – supplements are an optional extra.

Low levels of vitamin D have been linked to osteoporosis, depression, fibromyalgia, heart disease, high blood pressure, cancer and autoimmune conditions like MS.

As a result of our shorter days, lack of sunlight and cloudy skies, people living in the UK and Ireland have a high chance of being deficient in this crucial vitamin, especially in autumn and winter, so it is worth getting your levels tested.

Although there are some food sources for Vitamin D – like salmon, mackerel, sardines and eggs – the amount in food is minimal compared to that produced in the body from sun exposure. Most reports suggest supplementing around 2200iu a day to ensure your body has optimal levels.

Superfoods

Brassicas

The sulphurous vegetables classified as brassicas (also known as cruciferous vegetables) are some of the most nutritious foods on earth and include broccoli, cabbage, cauliflower, watercress, kale, kohlrabi, Brussels sprouts, rocket, turnip and purple-sprouting broccoli.

These apparently ordinary vegetables are in fact some of the most powerful ingredients in our veg box. They have the sulphur-based glucosinolates like isothiocyanates and indole-3-carbinol to thank for their smell, taste and health-promoting benefits. The active ingredients in these vegetables may provide some protection against cancer.

5. A high-strength probiotic

I like to add a high-strength probiotic to my supplement plan every so often. If you are feeling run down, your digestion is slightly off balance or if you have been prescribed an antibiotic, then a probiotic supplement could help rebalance your gut microbiome.

'What's the difference between a prebiotic and a probiotic?' is a question I get asked a lot, and my way of explaining it is to suggest that you imagine your gut like a field. The crops are your probiotics (good bacteria) and the fertiliser (organic of course!) is the growth medium or prebiotic. Prebiotics are commonly listed on the label as FOS or inulin.

When looking at probiotics there are two strains of bacteria that have been proven to be particularly effective. These are lactobacillus and bifidobacteria. Aim to choose a probiotic with at least 20 billion bacteria for an optimal dose.

Some other options to consider:

for digestive support	• digestive enzymes to help support your body to break down protein, fat and carbohydrate • milk thistle complex for liver support • probiotic to replenish good gut flora
for stress balance	• lemon balm and L-Theanine • magnesium • rhodiola or Siberian ginseng
to support immunity	• elderberry • zinc and vitamin C • echinacea • vitamin D
to balance sugar cravings	• chromium • cinnamon • manganese • B vitamins

Does your pee glow in the dark?!

If you are used to taking nutritional supplements, you know what I am talking about – the bright luminous yellow colour of your pee that comes soon after you have taken your multivitamin.

This is absolutely harmless and is simply a by-product of vitamin B2 (riboflavin) metabolism, although it can be a bit disconcerting if it catches you unawares!

Checklist – your suggested daily supplements

1. A good-quality multi-nutrient formula
2. Plant-based antioxidant
3. A high-strength fish oil
4. Vitamin D (if your levels are low)

Chapter Twelve

The Recipes

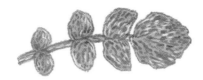

Breakfast salad bowl

Salad is not just for lunch or dinner. If you want to up your veggie intake with a nourishing breakfast, this recipe hits the spot.

> 2 eggs
> ½ avocado, peeled, stoned and sliced
> big handful of rocket or watercress
> 4 cherry tomatoes, halved
> ½ red pepper, sliced
> 40g (around 2 slices) smoked salmon

Bring a small pan of water to the boil and gently poach the eggs for about 2 minutes. Arrange the other ingredients on a plate or in a pasta bowl. Drain the eggs and place on top of the salad.

Enjoy as it is, or serve with some good sourdough bread or pumpernickel rye bread.

Overnight oats with pear and ginger

If you find it tricky to fit in all you have to do in the mornings, making breakfast the night before will save you time, energy and angst. I love overnight oats and find them a great way to make sure I get my day off to a healthy start. This recipe provides soluble fibre to support digestive health, ginger and omega-rich seeds which are anti-inflammatory, and the protein from the nuts and seeds will sustain you until lunchtime.

Serves 2
60g jumbo oats
1 pear, chopped
1–2 tsp grated fresh root ginger
1 dsp chia seeds
40g walnuts or hazelnuts
250ml milk of your choice

Place the oats and pear in an airtight container. Stir in the ginger, chia seeds and nuts. Pour over the milk, cover and store in the fridge overnight. You can add some natural yogurt and berries in the morning, or just eat it as it is. Sometimes I make enough to do a couple of days as the mixture will keep well in the fridge for 2–3 days.

Sugar-free nutty granola

Most commercial granolas are laden with sugar and vegetable oil. Not very healthy! This nutritious and delicious version is oil free and sugar free. Makes enough to do all week.

Makes 6–8 servings
100g jumbo oats
100g sunflower seeds
100g hazelnuts, crushed or roughly chopped
100g pumpkin seeds
1 tsp mixed spice

1 tsp ground cinnamon
sea salt
2 egg whites
juice of half a lemon
1 tbsp coconut nectar or maple syrup (optional)

Preheat the oven to 180°C/160°C fan/gas mark 4 and line a large baking tray with greaseproof paper.

Combine the dry ingredients in a large bowl with a pinch of salt.

Whisk the egg whites until they are fluffy in a separate bowl, and then fold them into the dry ingredients. Stir in the lemon juice and syrup (if you are using it).

Spread the granola mixture over the baking tray and bake for 40–45 minutes until lightly golden. As you near the end of the cooking time, check the granola every now and then to make sure it doesn't burn.

Allow to cool, then store in an airtight container, and enjoy with natural yogurt and berries.

Berry nutty shake

Packed with slow-release carbohydrate, plant-based protein and antioxidants, this shake is ideal as a post-workout recovery.

Serves 2
1 banana
500ml unsweetened almond milk
1 heaped dsp no-added-sugar peanut butter
1 dsp chia seeds
180g frozen berries
2 heaped dsp cacao powder

Put everything into your blender or smoothie maker, blitz and drink immediately.

Waldorf salad

A healthy version of the 1970s' favourite, this crisp, fresh salad is an ideal accompaniment to fish or chicken for lunch.

Serves 1–2 as a main course; 4 as a side dish
2–3 sticks celery, chopped
1 apple, cored and chopped
2 big handfuls of walnuts, crushed with the flat side of your knife

For the dressing:
1 tbsp natural yogurt
1 tsp Dijon mustard
1 tbsp apple cider vinegar
1 dsp extra-virgin olive oil
sea salt and freshly ground black pepper

Combine the celery, apple and walnuts in a bowl.
To make the dressing, mix all the ingredients together in a separate bowl and season.
Add the dressing to the rest of the ingredients, mix well and serve.

Fennel and orange salad

The refreshing combination of fennel and orange with a little mint is an ideal tonic for digestive health. Try it with whole baked trout (page 154) or roast chicken.

Serves 1 or 2 as a side dish
1 large orange
1 large fennel bulb, finely sliced
100g walnuts, crushed with the flat side of your knife
1 tbsp olive oil
a few sprigs of mint
sea salt and freshly ground black pepper

Cut the ends off the orange and set it flat on your chopping board. Use a small sharp knife to remove the skin and pith. Cut the orange into segments and cut each segment into 3 or 4 small pieces. Place in a bowl with any juice.

Add the finely sliced fennel and crushed walnuts. Drizzle with olive oil, add the mint and season well. This can be eaten on the day you make it, or will keep overnight in the fridge.

Super-greens sauce

I love this recipe because it packs a mighty nutritional punch. It is so versatile and can be served as a sauce with fish or chicken, or used as a salad dressing or dip. I tend to make it up, store in a Kilner jar in the fridge and use it over 2 or 3 days. It is one of those things that gets better over time, so I tend to make it a couple of hours before I want to use it.

80–100g organic rocket, watercress and spinach
60g fresh, soft green herbs like parsley, tarragon or basil (or a mixture)
2 tsp capers
3 tbsp good-quality olive oil
juice and zest of a lemon
sea salt and freshly ground black pepper

Whiz everything together in a blender or Nutribullet until it forms a smooth sauce. It will look like pesto.

Spinach, red pepper and cottage cheese frittata

Frittata is my go-to for a midweek lunch or dinner, and it's just as tasty eaten hot or cold. I love using this recipe to make mini frittatas to pop in my lunchbox with a salad. Make enough to do 2 or 3 days. You can make this recipe with almost any vegetables, depending on what's in your fridge or freezer and what's in season. Try making it with peas, broad beans, spinach and scallions in spring or summer, or broccoli, mushrooms, finely shredded kale and a little bit of chilli in the autumn or winter.

Serves 4–6
olive oil, for greasing
1 red onion, finely sliced
1 red pepper, sliced
100g spinach
6 eggs
300g cottage cheese
bunch of fresh parsley, chopped

To make a large frittata:
Preheat the oven to 180°C/160°C fan/gas mark 4. Lightly grease a 20cm square tin or lasagne dish.

Layer the sliced onion, peppers and spinach in the dish and place in the oven for 10 minutes to soften.

Whisk the eggs with the cottage cheese. Chop the parsley and add to the egg mixture.

Take the vegetables out of the oven and pour the egg mixture over. Bake for 20–25 minutes, or until just set. Leave to cool a little before cutting into slices and serving with a fresh green salad.

To make mini frittatas:
Preheat the oven to 180°C/160°C fan/gas mark 4. Lightly grease a 12-hole muffin tin.

Heat a little oil in a shallow pan over a medium heat. Cook the onion and pepper for a few minutes until the onion is softened. Add the spinach and cook until just wilted (about 2–3minutes). Mix in the chopped parsley and spoon into the muffin tray.

Whisk the eggs with the cottage cheese and divide evenly between the muffin holes.

Bake for 18–20 minutes, or until just set. Leave to cool a little before serving. These will store well in the fridge for up to three days.

Quinoa tabbouleh

Tabbouleh is a Middle Eastern salad packed with flavour and phytonutrients. I have replaced the traditional bulgur wheat with quinoa for even more nutrition. Serve with houmous and feta for a super-food meal.

I find the easiest way to measure quinoa is with a mug or cup and then add double the quantity of water for cooking.

Makes 4 servings
150g (about a mugful) of quinoa (or use a pack of ready-cooked quinoa)
6 scallions
60g flat-leaf parsley, chopped
30g fresh mint, chopped
100g pomegranate seeds
3 large tomatoes, finely chopped
1–2 cloves garlic, finely chopped
juice of a lemon
2 tbsp olive oil
sea salt and freshly ground black pepper

If you are using dried quinoa, place it in a saucepan with twice the volume of water and bring to the boil. Simmer for 10 minutes, then remove from the heat and leave to stand until all the water has been absorbed.

Place the scallions, parsley, mint, pomegranate seeds, tomatoes and garlic in a large bowl and mix together.

Place the quinoa in a sieve and rinse under cold running water. Drain well and add to the bowl with the rest of the ingredients.

Add the lemon juice and olive oil to the bowl. Season well, mix everything together thoroughly and serve.

Courgetti bolognese

A healthy twist on a family favourite. Using spiralised vegetables instead of pasta makes the meal lower GI and increases your vegetable intake. Courgetti works really well with bolognese and tastes so good you won't even miss the pasta. What's not to love?

Serves 4

1 tbsp olive oil or 1 dsp coconut oil

500g organic minced steak

1 large onion, finely chopped

4 cloves garlic, finely chopped

1 red pepper, chopped

2 sticks celery, finely chopped

1 large leek, trimmed and finely chopped

1 carrot, grated

1 can chopped tomatoes (400g)

1 tsp dried or fresh oregano

1 tbsp tomato puree

1 tbsp Worcestershire sauce

1 glass red wine

4 courgettes, spiralised or made into ribbons using a vegetable peeler

Parmesan cheese, grated

1 small bunch of basil

sea salt and freshly ground black pepper

Heat the oil in a large heavy-based pan over a medium heat. Add the mince and cook until lightly browned. Add the onion, garlic, red pepper, celery and leek and cook for 3 minutes.

Stir in the grated carrot, tinned tomatoes, tomato puree and oregano. Add the wine and Worcestershire sauce. Stir well, cover and allow to simmer for 30–40 minutes until the sauce has reduced and the vegetables are tender.

A few minutes before the bolognese is ready, heat a little olive oil in a wok and add the courgetti. Cook for a couple of minutes just to heat through – not too long or the courgetti will go mushy.

Season the bolognese and serve over the courgetti with a little Parmesan, some torn basil leaves and extra freshly ground black pepper.

Curry in a hurry

This curry is healthy fast food at its best. Make enough to do two nights for even more convenience.

Serves 4
1–2 tbsp tikka curry paste
1 onion, chopped
1 can chopped tomatoes (400g)
1 can chickpeas (400g), drained and rinsed
1 red pepper
1 green pepper
250g spinach
juice of half a lemon
sea salt and freshly ground black pepper

Heat the curry paste in a large non-stick pan. Once it starts to split, add the onion and cook for 2 minutes to soften. Tip in the tomatoes and allow to simmer for 5 minutes, or until the sauce has reduced. Add the chickpeas and vegetables, and season well, then cook for another couple of minutes.

Add the lemon juice, check the seasoning and serve with cauliflower rice (below).

Cauliflower rice

Home-made cauliflower rice is so fast, and as long as you cook it as soon as you prep it, you don't lose any essential nutrition along the way.

1 cauliflower, divided into florets
coconut oil

Simply break your cauliflower into florets and whiz in your food processor until it resembles rice or couscous. Don't over-blitz it. Stir-fry for a couple of minutes in a little coconut oil and it's ready to serve with your favourite home-made curry, chilli or stir-fry.

Rosemary, lemon and thyme chicken

Rosemary and thyme and incredibly rich in antioxidants and give this dish a lovely herby flavour. Make twice what you need and eat the leftovers for lunch tomorrow.

1 tbsp fresh rosemary, finely chopped
1 tbsp fresh thyme, finely chopped
4 cloves garlic, crushed or finely chopped
juice and zest of a lemon
2 tbsp olive oil
1 tsp Dijon or English mustard
sea salt and freshly ground black pepper
750g organic chicken thighs and drumsticks

Finely chop the rosemary, thyme and garlic. Add them to a large Ziploc bag with the lemon juice and zest, olive oil, mustard and seasoning, and mix well.

Place the chicken into the bag and make sure it's thoroughly coated in the marinade. Squeeze out as much air as possible, seal the bag and put it in the fridge to allow the chicken to marinade for 2 hours (or overnight).

When you are ready to cook, preheat the oven to 190°C/170°C fan/gas mark 5.

Pour the chicken and marinade on to a baking tray. Cook on the middle shelf of the oven for 35–40 minutes.

Serve with a fresh green salad and quinoa tabbouleh (page 151).

Whole baked trout

Trout is rich in omega-3 fats, and this way of cooking seals in the flavour.

Serves 2
2 whole trout, scaled, cleaned and gutted (ask your fishmonger)
2 sprigs rosemary
2 sprigs thyme
4 bay leaves
1 lemon, cut into wedges

olive oil
sea salt and freshly ground black pepper

Preheat your oven to 220°C/200°C fan/gas mark 7.

Place each trout on a large sheet of tinfoil and stuff the cavity with the herbs and lemon wedges. Drizzle with olive oil and season well. Seal the edges of the foil so that each piece of fish is now in its own parcel.

Bake for 20 minutes, or until the fish is cooked all the way through. Serve hot or cold.

Prawns with basil and tomato courgetti

This is one of my favourite fast recipes. Prawns are a great source of protein and also contain some omega-3 fats. The pink pigment in prawns is thanks to a powerful antioxidant called astaxanthin.

Serves 2
200g raw, peeled prawns
juice of a lemon
coconut oil
1 courgette, spiralised or made into ribbons using a vegetable peeler
1 red onion, sliced
handful of cherry tomatoes
1 red pepper, chopped
1 garlic clove, crushed and chopped
1 small bunch of basil
coconut oil
sea salt and freshly ground black pepper

Marinade the prawns in the lemon juice in a small bowl for a couple of minutes while you chop the vegetables.

Heat the coconut oil in your wok.

Stir-fry the prawns until they change to a pink colour. Add the onion and cook for a minute or so before adding the other vegetables. After another minute, tear in some fresh basil and season. Tuck in straightaway.

Chicken and orange tagine

Long slow cooking helps tenderise the chicken in this dish, making it easy to digest. With the turmeric, garlic, ginger and soluble fibre from the root vegetables, this dish is packed full of ingredients that are soothing and healing for your digestive system.

Serves 4–6

1 dsp coconut or olive oil
4–6 chicken thighs, skin on, bone in
4 carrots, chopped
1 large onion, chopped
1 sweet potato, peeled and chopped
4 garlic cloves, roughly chopped
a thumb-sized piece of ginger, grated
2 cinnamon sticks
1 tsp cinnamon
1 tsp turmeric
1 tsp cumin
1 tsp ground coriander
½ tsp dried chillies
2 sticks celery, chopped
1 red pepper, chopped
1 green pepper, chopped
1 can chopped tomatoes (400g)
500ml chicken stock
1 orange, chopped into 6–8 segments
1 can butter beans (400g), drained and rinsed
70g pitted green olives
200g fresh or frozen spinach
small bunch of flat-leaf parsley
sea salt and freshly ground black pepper

Preheat the oven to 200°C/180°C fan/gas mark 6.

Heat the oil in a large ovenproof pot on the hob and add the chicken, skin-side down. Cook until golden.

Add the carrot, onion, sweet potato, garlic and ginger and cook for 2–3 minutes. Stir in the spices and cook for a further couple of minutes. Add the celery, peppers, tomatoes, stock, orange, butter beans and olives.

Season well, cover and bake in the oven for 1 hour 20 minutes.

Before serving, remove the orange segments, take the chicken off the bone, and stir in the spinach and parsley.

Red cabbage and orange kraut

Inspired by my friend Dearbhla Reynolds from The Cultured Club, who specialises in all things fermented, this recipe was my first attempt at home-made kraut. This delicious combination is a fail-safe way to start making your own fermented food.

1 red cabbage, cored and finely shredded
sea salt
1 orange, finely sliced

Place the cabbage in a bowl with a good sprinkle of sea salt. Massage until the cabbage starts to get juicy. Leave to sit for 20–30 minutes.

Add the orange and massage the mixture again. By this stage it should be nice and juicy, with lots of water coming out of the cabbage.

Put the mixture into a 1-litre Kilner jar, pressing each handful down really firmly to reduce air pockets and increase juiciness. Place a weight on the top so all the cabbage and orange is submerged under the liquid.

Leave on a shelf for a few days. Do a taste test after 3–4 days and again after 7–8 days to see how your ferment is coming on.

You can eat when you like, but the longer you leave it, the more it ferments.

Proper chicken stock

Stock, or bone broth, has a high concentration of minerals, gelatin and collagen.

leftover chicken carcass
3 bay leaves
1 onion, roughly chopped
1 leek, trimmed and roughly chopped
2 large carrots, roughly chopped
2 sticks celery, roughly chopped
1 dsp apple cider vinegar

Place the chicken carcass in a large saucepan with the bay leaves, vegetables and apple cider vinegar. Cover with cold water until everything is submerged and bring to the boil. Skim off any fat or scum you see forming and simmer with the lid on for about 4 hours, topping up with water as necessary.

Pour through a sieve and allow to cool before refrigerating. It will keep in the fridge for up to a week or can be frozen.

Turmeric and ginger tea

This spicy tea, made with anti-inflammatory turmeric and ginger, is a perfect pick-me-up if you are feeling rundown or under the weather.

1 tsp ground turmeric
½–1 tsp ground ginger
½ tsp ground nutmeg
1 mugful water
freshly ground black pepper
honey, to taste

Place all the ingredients with a pinch of pepper in a small saucepan and simmer for 10 minutes. Strain and sweeten to taste with honey. Best served hot – to warm you from the inside out.

Coconut bites

… because every now and then everyone needs a sweet treat!

Makes 12–15
100g creamed coconut
2 tbsp coconut oil
100g unsweetened desiccated coconut
1 tsp vanilla extract
zest of a lemon
1 tbsp honey or coconut nectar syrup (optional)

Line a baking tray with cling film or baking parchment. Chop the creamed coconut into chunks and place in a small bowl over boiling water to melt, stirring occasionally.
Melt the coconut oil by placing the jar in a bowl of hot water for a few minutes.
Mix the desiccated coconut, melted coconut oil and melted creamed coconut together in a bowl. Stir in the vanilla extract, lemon zest and honey or syrup (if using).
Roll the mixture into small, bite-sized balls and place in the fridge for about 20 minutes.

Indulgent (but healthy) hot chocolate

Serves 1
1 tsp cacao powder
1 tsp vanilla extract (not essence)
250ml milk of your choice

Mix the cacao powder and vanilla extract together with a little of the cold milk in a mug to make a paste. Heat the rest of the milk gently in a saucepan, then pour it into the mug. Stir well and finish with a sprinkling of cacao powder or ground cinnamon.

Peanut and maca power balls

Maca is a Peruvian root renowned for its adaptogenic, adrenal-balancing effects.

Makes 12–15
2 tbsp smooth, no-added-sugar peanut butter
1 tbsp coconut flour
1 tbsp agave or coconut nectar syrup
1 tbsp maca powder
½ tsp vanilla extract (not essence)
30g dark chocolate (85 per cent cocoa solids)

Line a baking tray with cling film or baking parchment.

Mix the peanut butter, coconut flour, syrup, maca and vanilla extract in a bowl. Place the mixture in the fridge for 5–10 minutes. Melt the chocolate in a small bowl over hot water. Take the mixture out of the fridge, roll into bite-sized balls and dip into the melted chocolate. Place on the lined baking tray and put back into the fridge for 20 minutes or until you are ready to eat them.

Healthy chocolate mousse

A cheeky way to maximise your intake of good fats, soluble fibre and antioxidants.

1 ripe avocado
1 banana, peeled and sliced
1 tsp ground cinnamon
3 dsp raw cacao powder (or cocoa powder)
1 tsp vanilla extract
2 dsp coconut milk
handful of hazelnuts, to serve

Put the avocado flesh and the banana (leaving a few slices for decoration) into your food processor or blender with the other ingredients. Whiz until everything is well combined and serve with a topping of the reserved sliced banana and some hazelnuts.